FATHERING AND POVERTY

Uncovering Men's Participation in Low-Income Family Life

Anna Tarrant

T0256751

First published in Great Britain in 2021 by

Policy Press, an imprint of
Bristol University Press
University of Bristol
1-9 Old Park Hill
Bristol
BS2 8BB
UK
t: +44 (0)117 954 5940
e: bup-info@bristol.ac.uk

Details of international sales and distribution partners are available at
policy.bristoluniversitypress.co.uk

British Library Cataloguing in Publication Data
A catalogue record for this book is available from the British Library

ISBN 978-1-4473-4551-0 hardcover
ISBN 978-1-4473-4866-5 paperback
ISBN 978-1-4473-4868-9 ePub
ISBN 978-1-4473-4867-2 ePdf

Cover design: Robin Hawes.
Front cover image: iStock/Darren_russell
Bristol University Press and Policy Press use environmentally responsible
print partners.
Printed in Great Britain by CMP, Poole

I dedicate this book to my children, Lorelei and Wilf,

and my husband, Jamie.

Contents

List of figures and tables

Figures

Tables

List of abbreviations

FYF	Following Young Fathers
FYFF	Following Young Fathers Further
IGE	Intergenerational Exchange
MOC	mother of one's child
MPLC	Men, Poverty and Lifetimes of Care
QLR	qualitative longitudinal research

About the author

Anna Tarrant is Associate Professor in Sociology at the University of Lincoln and is a UK Research and Innovation Future Leaders Fellow (2020–24). Her research interests include men and masculinities, family life, the lifecourse and methodological developments in qualitative secondary analysis. Her current funded study, 'Following Young Fathers Further', is a qualitative longitudinal, participatory study of the lives and support needs of young fathers. She also edited *Qualitative Secondary Analysis* (2019, with Kahryn Hughes).

Acknowledgements

A sole-authored monograph, or indeed any academic output, is never an individual endeavour. I have so many people to thank for their support over the years; for helping to ensure the success of the Men, Poverty and Lifetimes of Care (MPLC) study, for championing me personally and for supporting the writing of this book. So here goes!

To the study participants: my thanks, first and foremost, must go to the participants of the MPLC study. This includes the professionals and organisations who generously gave their time and provided valuable insights about their work and the practice environments of which they are an essential part. I find myself constantly awed by the passion and drive shown by professionals who support families and individuals. I am always humbled by the knowledge and expertise you carry and are so willing to share so that things can change for the better. Thanks also to the 26 men who participated in interviews and to the attendees at the community centre who allowed me to be part of your everyday lives. You invited me into your worlds with great generosity and openness and expanded my view of the world. The care you show to your families is inspiring and I hope that, in your being given a voice through the pages of this book, your efforts are both appropriately acknowledged and supported.

To the study funder: the MPLC study was funded by the Leverhulme Trust Early Career Fellowship scheme between October 2014 and July 2018. When I discovered I had been awarded the funding I had already decided it was time to leave academia and was working for a charity. This funding brought me firmly back into academic life and put me back on a career path I could not even have dreamed of.

To the publishers: thanks to everyone whom I have worked with at Policy Press and to the reviewers of my book proposal and first book draft.

To those who supported the research: a huge thank you to Dr Ged Hall for helping me to design and run the knowledge-exchange workshop. To Professor Sarah Irwin, Dr Laura Davies, Dr Esmée Hanna, Dr Nick Emmel and Dr Carmen Lau-Clayton at the University of Leeds, who supported me with the qualitative secondary analysis work and were generous with your time and insights. I also take this opportunity to mention other colleagues whose work has strongly informed my own thinking. I am also honoured to call several of you close friends. Thanks to Dr Emily Cooper, Dr Sarah-Marie Hall, Dr Rachela Colosi, Dr Ana Jordan, Dr Mike Ward and Dr

Martin Robb. There are many more. Colleagues at the University of Lincoln who have also supported me and continue to do so to take my research ambitions forward include Linzi Ladlow, Dr Laura Way, Ben Handysides, Professor Stuart Humphries, Lyndsey Kemsley and Dr Paula Eves.

Thanks also to those of you who agreed to comment on early drafts of this book. To Dr Sarah-Marie Hall, Dr Steven Roberts, Dr Ana Jordan, Dr Yuliya Hilevych and Linzi Ladlow. Writing this book has been a challenge, not least because I wrote much of it during a pandemic. Your faith and guidance have undoubtedly strengthened my contribution and I value your input more than I can express.

I also write this book in memory of Professor Jacqui Briggs, who was tragically lost to cancer suddenly in July 2017. As Head of the School of Social and Political Sciences at the University of Lincoln, I will always remember you vividly for the passion, fairness and kindness you afforded to those around you. You are sorely missed.

Special mentions are essential for my inspirational mentors, Professor Bren Neale and Dr Kahryn Hughes. You have both taken me under your wing and seen something in me that has pushed me onwards and helped me to become the academic I am today. I hope that I am following in your footsteps by being simultaneously collegiate, intellectually generous and formidable. To Kahryn especially, while you started out as my MPLC study mentor, you have quickly become a trusted colleague and friend and our work together has been transformative for me, both personally and for my career. Thank you for always believing in me, for advising me, for pushing me onwards when things have been difficult and for being the most caring and genuine person I have ever had the privilege of knowing.

To my friends. Wherever I have lived, I have always found a 'bestie', those people who champion me, laugh with and at me, push me on and challenge me to think and do things differently. To Amy Elliott, Jenny Collyer, Miriam McDonagh, Anna Pattison, Emma Williamson and Harriet Samson-Bailey. I am honoured you have chosen me to be your friend.

To my family, my ever-constant source of love and support. You always keep me on track. To my mum and dad, Sally and Phil. My sisters and partners in crime, Katie and Claire. My lovely niece Sienna. My grandad, Andrew Porteous. To the Tarrant family, who welcomed me all those years ago. You have always made me feel at home as one of you.

To my children, Lorelei and Wilf. Lorelei, you were born less than a year before MPLC started. You are an epic and admirable combination of fierce, bright, passionate and assertive. You are also simultaneously caring, considerate and kind. You rocked my world when you were born and you continue to do so daily. As your own biography unfolds, know how much I admire you. I relish watching you flourish and grow. And to Wilf, my youngest born. You are boisterous, funny and utterly gorgeous. I love you both more than I can convey in words.

Most of all, this book is for my husband, Jamie. You are a constant source of love, laughter and happiness and have been from the moment we met. Your unwavering belief in me pushes me onwards. We've been together for 15 years and in that time your support, patience, thoughtfulness, humour and great music taste have inspired me the most. Thank you for all that you do and here's to many more festivals lugging the kids through mud!

Introduction: Fathering, poverty, families and policy

For children growing up in some of the poorest parts of the country, men are rarely encountered in the home or in the classroom. This is an ignored form of deprivation that can have profoundly damaging consequences on social and mental development. There are '*men deserts*' in many parts of our towns and cities and we urgently need to wake up to what is going wrong. (Fractured Families Report press release, Centre for Social Justice, 2013)

'From when I left my ex, I was paying [ex-partner] maintenance, but she was refusing to let me see [son from previous relationship] … my ex-partner, she's never worked and she's always sat on benefits, which then affected what happened to me, with the Child Support Agency[1] … What she did was, she took two part time jobs … they weren't legal jobs. The emphasis was then on me to grass her up for working on the side whilst at the same time being pursued for maintenance by the Child Support Agency. I couldn't convince them, because they saw me just as an *absent father* who was disgruntled and would say anything. Although I had four step-children, they dismissed [names of step-children with current partner Carolyn] and said that they, and they actually wrote to us … they said, "they do not count, you are an absent parent". It meant Carolyn was worse off and her children were worse off than before I moved in and I thought that was intolerable.' (Victor, aged 44, re-partnered, low-income father, interviewed for the Timescapes[2] Intergenerational Exchange study in 2008, Hughes and Emmel, 2011)

'Because you're young parents, you don't tend to get the respect. I mean, I remember a nurse coming in and saying to us, "oh, have you got a social worker coming in or something?" I turned round [and] just said, "I don't know why they'd be coming to see me! I didn't want to sort of be prejudiced against people but I think in the heat of the moment it just came out ... I'm not some scumbag that's just having kids willy-nilly, here there and everywhere. I'm not from the estates round here.'" (Tommy, aged 22, young father, interviewed in 2012 for the Timescapes Following Young Fathers study, Neale et al, 2015)

As these opening quotes illustrate, the relationship between fathering, poverty and policy is complex, contested and subject to multiple and often competing perspectives. Contrast policy discourses in the last decade, which tend to be constructed around simplistic, deficit narratives of absent fatherhood and fatherlessness like those promoted by the Centre for Social Justice, with rare accounts from men who are fathering in low-income families and there is an evident disconnect between the two. Why this might be has rarely been the subject of scrutiny or analysis.

In the context of the COVID-19 pandemic, which at the time of writing is both entrenching and exacerbating existing inequalities, with major impacts on low-income families (Patrick et al, 2020), on the gendered organisation of work and family life (Chung and van de Lippe, 2021), and on masculinities and fathering (Ruxton and Burrell, 2020; Tarrant et al, 2021a), attention to the evolving and intersectional relationships between fathering, poverty, families, and policy have become even more pertinent. This book seeks to explain why.

Drawing on evidence produced via a range of methodological strategies for a study called 'Men, Poverty and Lifetimes of Care' (MPLC), *Fathering and Poverty* seeks to redress and extend a limited and fragmented evidence base on low-income fatherhood, in a context in which myths of workless, absent and feckless fathers remain largely unchecked and unchallenged and rarely consider the complexities of men's lives or the broader patterns of care-giving in which they engage across the lifecourse. Our starting point, both for this chapter and for this book, is an exploration of the current state of debate in relation to contemporary knowledge and understanding of men's participation in low-income families, as a call for greater evidence and scrutiny of the realities of the contexts in which fathering on a low-income occurs.

'Dad deprivation': the current state of policy and public debate

Fears about the social causes and consequences of fatherless low-income communities are longstanding. Yet they notably intensified in debates and discussion following the summer of 2011, when the UK witnessed four days of rioting and protest across London and several major English urban centres. Provoked by a complex mix of socioeconomic factors (Ashe, 2014), but initially triggered by the death of 29-year-old Trey Duggan in Tottenham following a fatal shooting by police officers, the riots were indicative of a wider mood of discontent in the country at the time. Explanations for the rioting from those on the political left and right picked up on familiar themes and tropes (Featherstone et al, 2017). Despite the varied and multiple factors at play in driving young people to the streets, the troubles and disadvantages experienced by the young men from deprived localities who participated were expressed in public and political discourse as evidence of a toxic and dual 'crisis of masculinity' (Hearn, 1998; McDowell, 2003) and 'fatherlessness' (Williams, 1998). They were considered the outcome of 'dad deprivation' (Ashe, 2014) pervading many of Britain's low-income families and localities.

Echoing the sentiments expressed by the Centre for Social Justice, David Cameron, the then UK Prime Minister, made a speech on 15 August 2015 that explicitly linked the urban disorder with poor and absent parenting located in deprived neighbourhoods and localities. The emphasis for the blame was specifically placed on lone mothers who did not discipline their children and explicit reference was made to absent fathers and a lack of male role models, especially in the lives of boys and young men. Cameron said:

> 'I don't doubt that many of the rioters out last week have no father at home. Perhaps they come from one of the neighbourhood's where it's standard for children to have a mum and not a dad … where it's normal for young men to grow up without a male role model, looking to the streets for their father figures, filled up with rage and anger.'

As part of an enduring agenda about the negative social consequences of poor parenting and intergenerational cultures of worklessness, public discourses and policy debates encapsulated a complex constellation of societal concerns including criminality, violence and social disadvantage. A discourse of 'feral' parenting (De Benedictis, 2012) also emerged to describe an apparent 'underclass' of families thought to be residing in some of the UK's most deprived urban areas. Working-class men living in areas of social deprivation were constructed as uncaring, absent, feckless and/or disinterested in family life in a manner strongly infused with class stigmatisation (Tarrant and Neale, 2017a; see also Tarrant, 2021).

As noted by Ashe (2014: 652) in the aftermath of the riots, 'predictably, accounting for the riots became a point of discursive controversy as narratives about the moral irresponsibility of the participants and their parents vied with structural analyses for explanatory hegemony'. Indeed, in the years that followed, feminist researchers developed significant critiques of the ideologies and discourses directed at low-income families, identifying the classed and gendered assumptions on which they were based. Cameron's speech, for example, has notably attracted academic critique (for example, Harker and Martin, 2012; Jensen, 2018), not least because it so effectively consolidated media-led and political views of contemporary low-income families in the post-riot context, which individualised parenting and sustained a victim-blaming approach (Reynolds, 2020). In an analysis of his now infamous statement, Jensen (2018) argues that the power of Cameron's words lay in the way in which the key explanatory threads of fatherlessness and family breakdown carried the authority of common sense, were well rehearsed and said to need no evidence.

Following the riots, a wider social sciences scholarship unpicked how parent blame manifested predominantly as lone-mother blame (Allen et al, 2014; De Benedictis, 2012; Jensen, 2018), although precepts of 'good parenting' were extended to non-resident fathers as well (Jensen, 2018). The sophisticated and complex languages used to blame women were in no way matched in their application to fathers, but 'bad fathers' were politicised and presented as a special case where they were framed as distant, less capable and less burdened by the requirements of parenthood (Jensen, 2018; see also Brooks and Hodkinson, 2020). Notwithstanding the deficit language used to vilify individual parents and families, these discourses became foundational to the increasingly punitive welfare and family-policy reforms implemented under the auspices of austerity (De Benedictis, 2012; Quaid, 2018), the definitive policy approach of the entire decade since 2010 (see also Chapter 2). They also built on a historical legacy of media-perpetuated fears, stereotypes and pathologised ideas about families that have long existed. Even at the time of writing this book, policy debates that centre on why Black boys are more likely to be victims of the rising knife crime epidemic in many UK towns and cities (Reynolds, 2020), rather predictably blame Black mothers and posit boys' need for fathers and male role models as a ready solution (see BBC News, 2020; Sewell, 2019).

In the decade since 2010, a raft of academic research has examined the links between gender, poverty and parenting in low-income families and communities from the perspectives of women and single mothers, women engage most in the 'non-economic' work of social reproduction (for example, Ridge, 2009; Millar and Ridge, 2009; Greer Murphy, 2019; Reynolds, 2020), and have been disproportionately affected by austerity policies. Men's experiences of family and parenting in contexts of disadvantage and under the conditions of recent and rapid socioeconomic transformation remain under-researched (Ridge, 2009; Tarrant, 2021). Furthermore, the character of men's absence from family lives, while often posited as a key cause of myriad contemporary social problems, is rarely problematised. Concerns about father absence and fatherlessness are underscored by an ongoing set of interrelated questions about the changing roles of men in society (as providers, citizens and role models) and policy and popular representations of families experiencing persistent poverty. Yet questions still remain. Why do marginalised men in low-income contexts continue to evoke such moral condemnation in the popular and dominant imagination? If men are not present in family or community contexts, where are they? Poverty research suggests that men are more likely to become socially isolated through a loss of employment and familial and community ties (Bennett and Daly, 2014). This can make it difficult for them to consider themselves in the context of family ties. However, the likelihood of a complete severance of interdependencies and family relations for all men seems implausible. If men are present in families, why are they absented and how do deficit attitudes and stereotypes work to sustain assumptions of their absence, especially from low-income contexts? An interrogation of the complexities of contemporary constructions of low-income fatherhood and their premise on binary conceptions of absence and presence, begins to offer some insight here.

Contemporary fatherhoods: Unpicking father absence and presence

As Dermott (2008) has argued, modern fatherhood is an intriguing topic of study that sparks polarised opinions both within the academy and beyond. It is affected by two trends simultaneously; increasing rates of parental break-up whereby fathers are non-resident and reside in different households from their children, and an increased emphasis on paternal involvement in the lives of young children (Skevik, 2006). Interpretations of these processes have resulted in a tendency to collapse into binary thinking around questions of father absence and presence (or involvement) and moral discourses that categorise 'good' and 'bad' fathers, revealing a conflict at the centre of societal expectations for men. Outlining what has been described as the 'two faces' and modern paradox of fatherhood (Furstenberg, 1998), social historian Joanne Bailey (2010: 267–8) neatly captures the deep and inherent societal confusion that characterises the role of men in family life today. She notes:

> the media judges how movie stars, celebrity sportsmen and politicians perform as fathers. Fiction and film explore fatherhood, and politicians and 'think-tanks' deplore failing and absent fathers. Our society admires what sociologists call the 'involved' father: emotionally accessible, participating in his children's routine activities and sharing in their care. At the same time law, policy and popular expectation defines a good father as an effective breadwinner. Social scientists expose the paradox at the centre of these ideals of fatherhood, which require high levels of involvement in children's lives while simultaneously demanding financial support through engagement in a workplace that promotes a 'long hours' culture.

Bailey's quote points to an ambivalence around men as carers and a proliferation of conflicting representations of fathers in popular culture that perpetuate a vivid sense of crisis at the heart of the paternal role (Freeman, 2003). A question that industrialised societies continually grapple with is whether and to what extent the absence of fathers is problematic.

Certainly, the enduring prevalence of concerns around the role of parenting in low-income communities overlaps with those around men and their involvements in the care of children as 'hot' topics that continue to be debated and discussed in many industrialised countries (Dermott, 2008; Robb, 2019). As the opening quote of this chapter demonstrates, fears about the ostensible absence of fathers from families and more generally from a range of social institutions including childcare settings, schools and family support services have retained their prominence in public debates and on political agendas (Tarrant and Ward, 2017). As demonstrated in the aftermath of the riots, these discourses locate the rising prevalence of non-resident fatherhood as a 'crisis of fatherlessness', thought to be specific to an alleged underclass. The idea that an 'underclass' of people exists, namely 'people at the bottom of the heap, structurally separate and culturally distinct from traditional patterns of "decent" working-class life' (MacDonald, 1997: 1), has become an increasing, if widely contested, idea in the two decades since 2000. These discussions stress that men's alleged fecklessness and the increased power attained by mothers through their greater access to welfare benefits (Featherstone, 2013) are responsible for the lack of male role models in the lives of boys. As part of an intergenerational repertoire, 'crisis of fatherlessness' and 'fatherless society' discourses are frequently invoked as explanatory factors in young men's expressions of discontent, their investments in violence, long-term unemployment (Morgan, 2003) and inability to meet societal expectations of masculinity.

The idea that contemporary families are experiencing multiple crises and that societies are becoming increasingly fatherless appeals to policy makers, commentators and politicians and is frequently preferred as an explanation for a range of societal ills (see Mann and Roseneil, 1994; Lammy, 2011; Mahadevan, 2011; Ashe, 2014; Featherstone et al, 2017). Especially prominent in the 1990s in the US, for example, fatherlessness was identified as *the* major social issue of the time. Citing Blankenhorn's near-apocalyptic, social conservative warning of an encroaching fatherless America, Baskerville (2004: 485) notes that nearly every major social pathology can be linked to children from fatherless homes. This includes: 'violent crime, drug and alcohol abuse, truancy, unwed pregnancy, suicide, and psychological disorders – all correlating more strongly with fatherlessness than with any other single factor, surpassing even race and poverty'. These are also international concerns. In South Africa, for example, there is significant empirical evidence of men's absence from households, which has been linked in part to specific cultural, customary and social practices, to migrant labour systems and to the impacts of the AIDS pandemic (Mavungu Eddy et al, 2013). Absent fatherhood here is often equated with lack of financial provision but has been critiqued for seriously underestimating men's financial and emotional supports for children (Richter and Morrell, 2006; Madhavan et al, 2010). In these perspectives, father absence is interpreted as low paternal involvement and financial provisioning and the product of men's lack of motivation to meet their parental obligations, namely breadwinning. These assumptions are replicated in policy contexts that understand poverty to be a consequence of poor life-style choices rather than the outcome of the social and economic barriers that men may face or the race and class inequalities that undermine them (Randles, 2018).

A cursory look at the national statistical picture in the UK broadly offers support for increasing rates of men's absence and non-residence from households, the main indicator of fatherlessness. According to recent statistics, 2.9 million children are living in lone-parent families in the UK, of which 90% are headed by women (Office for National Statistics, 2019); 1.1 million children are growing up without a father at home, at an estimated cost of £51 billion a year (Centre for Social Justice, 2017; Marriage Foundation, 2018); and 76% of young men in prison in England and Wales also reported growing up with an absent father (Prison Reform Trust, 2013). This evidence is often interpreted with pessimism, alongside concerns about the burden of the costs of family breakdown and dysfunctionality to the public purse. Family breakdown is thought to constitute one of five causal pathways to family poverty, alongside educational underachievement or failure, worklessness, addiction and serious personal debt (Centre for Social Justice, 2016). It therefore has high economic and social costs to society and, as noted earlier, is often connected to several key pathologies in young boys and men with potential for long-term effects.

Notable bodies of academic scholarship further underscore the case for the prevalence and pernicious outcomes of father absence, which are interpreted in the context of changes in family structures and couple relationships. American scholars McLanahan et al (2013) note the long tradition of sociological research, for example, that has examined its causal effects. They begin by identifying the relevance of questions of father absence, first to family sociologists and family demographers because of what it can be said to say about changes in contemporary family structures and family processes, and second to scholars of inequality and mobility because of what it can be said to say about how disadvantage is transmitted intergenerationally within families. A particular focus of these debates has been the immediate and longitudinal impacts of divorce and family breakdown on the economic and social-emotional well-being of children. This research evidences a range of adverse outcomes for children living apart from their biological fathers across multiple domains including education, mental health, family relationships and labour market outcomes, relative to children who grow up in ostensibly more stable family contexts (McLanahan et al, 2013). Children with absent fathers are also more likely to be economically disadvantaged (Edin and Kissane, 2010). Yet while family breakdown is influential in children's development, it is worth noting that not all families that experience breakdown produce problem children and not all children who experience problems have experience of conflict or the loss of primary paternal figures (Hollway, 2006).

The case for pessimism about the implications of family change and fatherlessness is also implicitly underscored by strong evidence confirming a correlation between the presence and involvement of men in family contexts and its immense value for them, their children, their partners and society (Featherstone, 2009; Carlson and Magnuson, 2011; Levtov et al, 2015; Morrell et al, 2016). Models of engaged and involved fatherhood are visibly promoted as the new cultural imperative (Miller, 2010a; Dermott and Gatrell, 2018) and include expectations that men provide for the physical needs of their children, as well as psychological support and moral guidance. Higher rates of paternal involvement in care are thought to correlate with parental relationship stability (Norman et al, 2018), and it is increasingly accepted that men's equitable and non-violent engagements in caregiving are important (Levtov et al, 2015). Among a range of reported benefits, there is consensus that father involvement influences the child's well-being and their social and educational development (Lamb, 2010; Cabrera et al, 2014; Poole et al, 2016; Richards Solomon, 2017). Women may feel empowered to enter the labour market and experience improved health, education and relationship outcomes (Levtov et al, 2015), and fathers also report improved physical and psychological health, including greater confidence and satisfaction in family life (Rosenberg and Wilcox, 2006). The intergenerational transmission of father involvement also has potential to positively influence how future generations share childcare and employment (Bartova and Keizer, 2020). The extent to which the ethos of father involvement remains more of an ideal than it is being realised in practice, however, is unpacked in more detail in Chapter 3.

There are other, counter arguments to consider here, including critiques that have been raised to suggest that dominant policy discourses are not the most effective way of explaining and understanding the complexities and diversities of men's lived experiences in low-income families and communities. There is evident need for some balance in terms of how existing evidence is interpreted, as well as the extent to which individual men and families can be fully held responsible for, and positioned as, the main causal factor for many of the complex social troubles that are ascribed to them. As Featherstone et al (2017) note, these discourses can only ever offer a simplified solution to otherwise complex social problems. This line of argumentation is taken forward next.

The absent presence of low-income men

When subject to interrogation, the empirical and intellectual basis for the existence of fatherless societies and absent fathers is much less easy to sustain. Rather, men's perspectives about low-income family life represent an absent presence in these debates overall. By this I mean that they are simultaneously hyper visible in representational contexts (such as media and policy discourse) yet absent according to the statistical picture, which focuses predominantly on their non-residence from households as biological fathers rather than on the complexities and dynamics of their family lives, identities and relationships.

The presence of low-income men is perhaps most evident in crisis rhetoric. In temporal perspective it is evident that heightened anxieties about the crisis of masculinity and linked crises of fatherlessness are far from novel. Despite years of sustained critique, masculinities in crisis rhetoric has proven to be remarkably durable, so much so that Roberts (2018) argues that scholars have become obligated to 'problematise the notion of crisis, while still recognising this rhetoric as an important contextual backdrop to empirical findings'. While the empirical focus of this book is low-income fathers rather than young working-class boys, it also endeavours to do the same. Both crises, of masculinity and of fatherlessness, are often presented as if they are new because they ostensibly explain the implications of unprecedented socioeconomic change (see Jordan, 2020a) with consequences for the lifecourse transitions and trajectories of boys and fathers. Yet as demonstrated by the example of the urban riots they also emerge cyclically and at specific times of social crisis, albeit with new languages and iterations. While the recent contextual conditions that affect change in men's lives, including the decline of heavy industry and manufacturing, women's increasing participation in the labour market and the relative underachievement of boys in education, are undoubtedly realities of life today for some men, the plausibility of the crisis and extent to which they constitute a crisis is still open to debate and discussion (Roberts, 2018). Certainly while men may be experiencing increased role insecurity and there are costs of masculinity for some men more than others, gendered structures continue to disadvantage women as a group more than men as a group (Jordan, 2020a).

A sensitive, intersectional analysis of masculinities is therefore important for understanding how and to what extent men's lives are contoured by wider structural processes and are either enabled or constrained by the material and social resources available to them (see Chapter 3). Reaching their height in the late 1990s, oversimplified media and political representations and discourses of crisis have been most critiqued for positioning boys and men as a homogeneous group and for espousing ideas of a singular, homogeneous masculinity (Maguire, 2020). They noticeably accrue to boys living in families in deprived localities and to men who 'father from the margins' (Abdill, 2018). While policy concerns are often expressed in relation to the impact of men's absence on boys, they also betray anxieties about lone-female headed households and typically target boys from working-class and Black and minority ethnic backgrounds, a population that represents the dominant prototype for the absent father (Reynolds, 2009). Thus, while cultural commentaries of masculinities in crisis superficially refer to a generic category of 'boys' and 'fathers', it is typically minoritised, working-class men, living in stigmatised places, who embody many of the 'troubles' described (Tarrant et al, 2015; Ward et al, 2017). Contemporary social portrayals of marginalised fathers are therefore often sensationalised because they are underscored by negative, stigmatising and discriminatory attitudes towards those experiencing poverty.

Conflicts at the heart of contemporary fatherhood are therefore explained in part by the intersecting inequalities that underscore representations of 'good' and 'bad' dads and wider perceptions of their family participation. In conceptual terms, involved fathers are more readily associated with 'good fathering' and 'poor fathers' with the working classes and deficit situations where involved fatherhood is thought to be less achievable (Gillies, 2009; Earley, 2017). In the current ideological and cultural context, images of 'good', involved, caring and hands-on fatherhoods (Braun et al, 2011) abound. However, they typically reflect middle-class values and biases (Klett-Davies, 2010) and an externally generated and idealised construct of fatherhood associated with men who are employed, partnered and ostensibly invested in the nurturance of their children. Non-resident and working-class fatherhoods, through their association with unemployment, poor economic provisioning and/or residence in different households are considered dysfunctional and irresponsible, despite ever-increasing diversity in family forms and experiences. Men who do not fulfil the expectations of involved fatherhood (or at least are perceived not to) are more vulnerable to being stereotyped, pathologised and blamed for failing their children (Henwood and Procter, 2003).

This discursive absenting is re-enforced by limited empirical engagement with men in low-income families or contexts. There is limited evidence to suggest there is any divergence in practices for fathers in different class contexts (Dermott and Pomati, 2016), although, as argued, research with low-income fathers is less developed than research with their more-resourced counterparts. Roberts (2018) also cautions that working-class masculinities are often inadvertently portrayed in pessimistic terms in academic research as well, enforced by a preoccupation with the problematic and spectacular elements of masculinity in ways that misrepresent more beneficial trends. Questions of father absence and presence are consequently delineated by class inequalities, whereby father presence is considered the preserve of middle-class fathers and families, and absence the preserve of men who are marginalised or deprived.

Noteworthy critiques have also been developed of the theoretical sophistication of the male role model discourse (Tarrant et al, 2015; Robb et al, 2018) as a gendered and intergenerational discourse on which father absence is premised. Underscored by a simplistic and reductive social learning model of gender identity and development, these discourses conceal the significance of other family dynamics in their simplistic and unitary emphasis on gender and processes of gender socialisation. The assumption that young men straightforwardly mimic the behaviours of their fathers or of other adult men and that gendered identities and practices are transmitted intergenerationally without transformation or change has been largely debunked by theoretical arguments that masculinities are plural, multifaceted and contextually specific (see Chapter 3). Policy and practice responses that are premised on the male role model discourse have also been appraised for assuming the primacy of the ascribed biological father. In a robust critique of the 'responsible fatherhood' programme in the US, for example, which is premised on such assumptions, Randles (2020) illustrates its promotion of a discourse of 'father essentiality' which suggests that fathers offer uniquely masculine roles that are essential to child development. These strategies often rely on an empirically unfounded rationale for father involvement, which, Randles argues, also individualises fatherlessness. Her insightful analysis demonstrates how racism, class and patriarchy intersect and reciprocally shape government parenting programming in ways that impact on the identities of marginalised men who are fathers (Randles, 2020) and obscure the efforts of other family members.

Anxieties raised about lone-mother households and absent fathers in the UK betray a comparable set of concerns and assumptions. The significant roles of mothers and other women in developing boys' identities and capacities to care, for example, are absented by these discourses. Recent evidence highlights the significant contributions that mothers and grandmothers make to the support of their sons and grandsons, particularly in low-income localities (McDowell, 2014;

Robb et al, 2018). As McDowell (2014) observes, in the context of the increasingly irregular and casual work characterising austerity that has replaced the nine-to-five labour on which manual employment was dependent, many young working-class men are now reliant on their mothers to establish a routine for them, representing a 'new sexual contract'. Research on gay and lesbian parenting also demonstrates few adjustment issues in children who grow up in non-heterosexual families without a father or mother figure (Segal, 2006). These findings illustrate the limits to gender as the sole explanatory framework and instead signal that couple households are more of a protective factor in the current economy. Positioning involved fathers as the solution therefore denies complexity in men's lives, devalues the essential role of women in social reproduction and even more problematically, may obscure some of the dangers that men may pose to families (Featherstone, 2009).

Linked to this, the absenting of men has been observed and problematised in child protection contexts, where men are often discounted because they are described by women either as absent or much too present. In their analysis of case notes based on accounts of family life by women and children in Canada, Brown et al (2009) identify men in families whom they describe as 'manufactured ghosts'. Here they refer to men who are mentioned, exist and are relevant in family contexts but are rarely seen in support contexts. Using case notes generated predominantly with women as data, they render visible a series of rotating fathers. This includes men who are absent from households but who still play active roles in their children's lives, or men who are scarcely acknowledged by women because they cannot, or choose not to, identify them. In these cases, father presence, rather than absence, produces negative consequences that are linked to the dangers of abuse and the control of women. In these ways, the vilification of lone-parent households, which are predominantly headed by women, often contributes further harms to women by obscuring their own efforts towards their families. Concerns have been raised, for example, that men may use arguments that children need a biological father to pursue anti-feminist aims that return women's dependence on men or reduce their autonomy (Richter and Morrell, 2006). Also obscured here are the wider sets of familial interdependencies that children may be situated within and engage in across households.

Judith Stacey (1998) interprets these dynamic processes not as a decline of family life but as a transformation of family structures, such that women now have increased choices to leave abusive or neglectful partners or husbands behind. The men who remain, she suggests, are more likely to be involved in family contexts in richer, more meaningful ways. Stacey's feminist intervention highlights how wider societal and political anxieties about men often also carry unarticulated anxieties about changes in the lives of women (Tarrant et al, 2015). Additionally, overemphasis on the prevalence of fatherless families also obscures those international contexts where men are often required to take on single-parent roles and tasks because there are high rates of female absence because of migration, as is the case for Ukraine, Slovakia and Romania (van der Gaag et al, 2019).

As these wide-ranging critiques demonstrate, the concept of absence (and presence as a corollary) is complex, variable and problematic. Meanings of absence are often used interchangeably and refer to any combination of *physical* absence of fathers from the household, *emotional* distance from children and/or *economic* absence, involving the relinquishment of financial provision (Dermott, 2008). While there are certainly a decreasing number of children residing in the same households as biological fathers in the UK (Poole et al, 2016), patterns of non-resident fatherhood are a consequence of changing family forms, increasing prevalence of divorce, remarriage and the emergence of reconstituted families where men become stepfathers (Allen and Daly, 2002). Popular and policy assertions tend to conflate the idea that fathers who live with their children support them, but those who do not live with them do not (Madhavan et al, 2010). As demonstrated by Bailey's (2010) earlier quote, however, the relationship between a father's physical location and the direct time and effort they invest in their children and in their family lives is not straightforward. Co-residence is therefore problematic as a measure of father presence and involvement (Madhavan et al, 2010).

Alternative stories?

To address the empirical absence of men in low-income contexts, I return again now to the accounts of Tommy and Victor, whose narratives were presented alongside the contemporary policy discourses used to commence this chapter. These men were interviewed for two qualitative longitudinal, sociological research studies conducted against the backdrop of rapid socio-economic change linked to the 2008 global economic crisis. Intergenerational Exchange (IGE) and Following Young Fathers (FYF) were connected to the Timescapes programme of research which provided unique evidence and insights into the diverse character of family life and the lived experiences of individuals at key stages of the lifecourse including through the economic downturn of

2008–9 (Edwards and Irwin, 2010; Neale and Holland, 2012). Briefly, IGE examined the longitudinal dynamics of low-income family life as experienced by grandparents residing in one low-income locality (Hughes and Emmel, funded 2006–2010). FYF explored the parenting journeys and support needs of young fathers aged 25 and under (Neale et al, 2015, funded and ran from 2010, for the first two years with ESRC Timescapes funding and then with separate ESRC funding from 2012). Both studies engaged with men from under-researched low-income families and communities. Secondary analysis of these datasets as part of the MPLC study was foundational to the design of a new empirical phase of research rooted in men's real concerns and lived experiences.

Narratives like those expressed by Tommy and Victor are rarely heard in social commentary today and have rarely been subject to depth analysis by researchers. In each of these relatively small excerpts, both men, both of whom were living on a low-income at the time they were interviewed and were ostensibly young to be a parent and grandparent, respectively, illustrate how men in low-income contexts negotiate and seek to disrupt public images of absent and feckless fathers. Their narratives demonstrate acute awareness of the ways in which they are talked about and thought of in public, practice and political arenas – images that they seek to distance themselves from on reflection about their perceptions of themselves, of others and their own family experiences. Young father Tommy strenuously dissociates himself from 'other' young fathers from local estates, whom he perceives, albeit reflexively, to be morally suspect, incapable and subject to surveillance by social workers and other health professionals. Similarly, grandfather Victor explicitly separates himself from the absent-father label imposed by the Child Support Agency in their requirements to enforce the payment of child maintenance. For Victor, as a man who holds multiple familial generational identities and positions as a father, stepfather, step-grandfather and foster carer, providing extensive and extended care and support both within and across several households, this kind of positioning is untenable.

Analyses of these contrasting accounts suggest that in a context where politicians, the media and policy think-tanks deplore absent fathers, the men they purport to represent distance themselves from such representations. At the very least, the narratives of Tommy and Victor indicate alternative trajectories for men in low-income families that are often obscured by the policy rhetoric of a fatherless society and the assumed prevalence of uncaring men and feckless families. Their repetition of ostensibly common-sense and widely held beliefs that are subtly reinforced by representations in the media and in political commentary are important because they are influenced by the dominant imagination (Alexander, 1998, cited by Hopkins, 2006). As Hopkins (2006) notes, understanding how masculinities (and in this book, those associated with the fatherhoods of low-income men) are socially constructed is important because they are given life by their articulation. More significant, though, is the value of generating rich, qualitative evidence about the lived experiences of men in these contexts. At present, observations of different forms of family participation by a diverse constituency of fathers and male adult carers are often rendered invisible through the very construction of men as absent. This is an argument now turned to in the remainder of the chapter to carve out a rationale for a more detailed sociological account of men's family lives and responsibilities in low-income families and contexts.

The absence of low-income fathers in qualitative research

Despite the reproduction of dichotomous discourses around loving or deadbeat dads in popular culture (Freeman, 2003) and policy contexts, fathers living in low-income family contexts are rarely given a voice in social sciences research. Notwithstanding evidence of the high prevalence of fatherless households, qualitative evidence that foregrounds the lived experiences and perspectives of men themselves is certainly lacking. In a rare review of research about fathers of Black Caribbean heritage in the UK (Fatherhood Institute, 2010), for example, a number of methodological blindspots are identified that are often replicated in research about low-income fathers more generally. These include issues of drawing on limited samples from socially excluded, inner-city communities; failing to account for age and social disadvantage; failures to acknowledge the extent of father involvement by non-resident fathers; and, as Segal (1990) suggests, ignoring the substantial involvement in childcare of other adult male family members.

As Segal (2006) notes, it has been difficult to consider the diversity of ways that men engage in care and invest in their family identities. Yet as part of an important critique of the resurgent absent father trope and its application to non-resident Black fathers, Reynolds (2010) asks provocatively, 'are we truly to believe that … there is a complete absence of male family members in these children's lives? What about the step-fathers, uncles, grandfathers, brothers, and male cousins, who often perform the fathering role in the absence of the biological father?'

Here, she draws attention to the significance of wider familial dynamics and generational identities that men may simultaneously hold, as well as the potential of men's engagements as social fathers. 'Social fathering' is an expanded definition of fatherhood that incorporates anyone, from 'a male sibling who is standing in for an absent or a deceased father, a grandfather, an older male family member, or an unrelated man who undertakes childcare' (Morrell et al, 2016: 82). According to Collier and Sheldon (2008) and Featherstone (2009), definitions of fathers are also delineated by status. Featherstone (2009) argues that men do not become fathers until they assume responsibility for a child, either social, legal or biological. Collier and Sheldon (2008) define social fathers as those who assume responsibilities with no legal or biological basis. Informed by these diverse definitions of fathers, this book adopts an inclusive approach that recognises male fathering and caregiving that occurs in a range of circumstances, whether formally or informally ratified. The complex biological, social and legal factors that determine men's experiences of parenting and caregiving (Philip et al, 2020) are also incorporated.

While it is apparent that contemporary social portrayals of low-income fathers homogenise men who are disadvantaged by their class, race, age or other intersectional inequalities, the veracity of these ideas is compounded by the lack of qualitative engagement with their fathering and familial experiences. This paucity of evidence is not just specific to fatherhood research. It is also notable across the three main thematic areas of this book and attests to the kinds of questions that researchers ask and the analytical lenses researchers adopt to understand fatherhood, poverty and family dynamics. A more detailed synthesis of these literatures is conducted in Chapters 2 and 3 to further elaborate these knowledge gaps and address blind spots in each set of debates, but they are considered briefly here.

Despite growing awareness of family diversity and the increasing complexity of fatherhoods (Lee, 2008), knowledge of fathering is predominantly based on the experiences of men who are transitioning to parenthood for the first time (Dermott and Miller, 2015), are securely involved in family life as secondary carers (for example, Dermott, 2008; Miller, 2010a; Doucet, 2011) or are stay-at-home fathers, often by choice (Chesley, 2011; Richards Solomon, 2017), and consequently resourced in a way that enables them to adhere to the ideological determinants of 'engaged fatherhood' (Miller, 2010a). Conceptually, understanding of the extent of gendered transformation in the division of employment and informal care work within families is therefore based predominantly on participant samples with materially similar experiences (Rao, 2020). The radical potential for empowering and transformative practices of masculinity to emerge among marginalised men and fathers and from sites or positions of marginality is also often overlooked in academic discourse and is only recently gaining much-needed attention in the context of discussions about working-class boys and young men (Elliott, 2020; Roberts and Elliott, 2020).

Neither has there been any sustained attempt in poverty research or the family poverty sub-field to explore men's experiences of parenting or providing care in low-income families in the UK context. To date, there has been limited sociological engagement and theorisation about the diverse biographies of young adult men in low-income localities, beyond the educational and economic facets of their transitions to adulthood (for example, MacDonald, 1997; Ward, 2015a; McDowell, 2017). Furthermore, the longitudinal and relational processes of deprivation that marginalise men, over time, both in and sometimes from family life are rarely examined. Family poverty research tends to prioritise women's experiences of social reproduction in low-income contexts or the interpersonal dynamics of poverty among couples (Goode and Waring, 2011; Demey et al, 2013 and see Chapter 2 for a more detailed review). There has been some consideration of how children experience family poverty too (Ridge, 2013). A notable feature of these contemporary disciplinary sub-fields that are relevant to an understanding of men's experiences in low-income contexts is that empirical engagement with marginalised and low-income fathers is often either partial or accessed implicitly via the accounts of others, namely women and children.

Despite being relatively fledgling areas of research, there have been some recent and notable additions to the evidence base. Several international studies of young and low-income fatherhoods are of note here, conducted in advanced industrialised countries like the UK and the US. In the UK, research on young fatherhood is notably based on the experiences of young, predominantly white men (Henwood et al, 2010; Neale et al, 2015); US-based research has also explored the racial dimensions of men's experiences of family in low-income contexts (Waller, 2002; Edin and Nelson, 2013; Roy et al, 2015; Abdill, 2018). Knowledge about the experiences of marginalised fathers is also apparent in research that considers men's engagements with social services and court proceedings (Maxwell et al, 2012; Philip et al, 2020) and in research exploring the role of dads' groups and support for men in low-income communities (for example, Dolan, 2014; Robertson et al, 2018; Tarrant and Neale, 2017b; Hanna, 2018). These research interests reflect when men in low-income contexts are most likely to become visible to researchers. More generally, however, relatively little work has been carried out with men who occupy marginal spaces in society (Haywood and Johannsson, 2017).

Overall, the lack of detailed qualitative research about men's family lives, responsibilities and family participation is problematic because it serves to perpetuate the impression of their absence. The paradox therein is that heightened policy and media concern is set against a limited and fragmented evidence base (Neale and Patrick, 2016). Notwithstanding the evident need to address the empirical neglect of the lived realities of fathers and wider male family members and their participation in low-income family contexts, there is also a clear need for new terms of debate and discussion and a renewed focus on the ways in which men themselves risk being deprived of family life in a context that individualises and chastises them rather than supports and champions when they have positive contributions to make.

Researching the family participation of men in low-income contexts

Funded by the Leverhulme Trust Early Career Fellowship scheme (award number ECF-2014-228, October 2014–July 2018), MPLC sought to address these wider societal concerns about fathers and low-income families by foregrounding the lived experiences of fathers and adult male carers in low-income families. In so doing, it sought to explore the complex relationship between fathering, poverty and policy through men's own accounts of their care responsibilities, support needs and patterns of care across the life course. As a sociologically informed study, MPLC therefore contributes a more comprehensive understanding of men's experiences of low-income contexts in a way that is less hijacked by the anxieties that manifest in public debate and that serves to amplify or even deny complex social problems.

A combination of interview, ethnographic and participatory visual methods were employed for the MPLC study to generate up-close, personal accounts of men's lives and trajectories. This design was premised on a micro-dynamic approach to researching the social world that aims to generate an 'intimate movie' and moving picture of the lives of individuals (Neale, 2019). Capturing and uncovering the micro-dynamics of men's lifecourses via socially constructed accounts of their lived experiences and life journeys both across time and place (Neale, 2019) also aimed to significantly shift debate beyond the static and polarised constructions of men's involvement in family life that are currently premised on snapshot and binary determinants of absence and presence, as described earlier.

Informed by a theoretical anchoring in qualitative longitudinal research (QLR), analysis of existing qualitative longitudinal data (Tarrant 2017; Tarrant and Hughes, 2019) and the intention to build a fuller picture of low-income family life and men's lived experiences and care responsibilities, the MPLC study took a lifecourse perspective and sought to consider how different aspects of help, support and care feature in the everyday relations of men in different familial generational[3] positions but similar socioeconomic locations (see Appendix 1 for participant sample). The unique empirical contribution of the book therefore is an analysis of semi-structured life-journey interviews with fathers and adult male carers at different stages of the lifecourse with diverse sets of caring responsibilities, family configurations and familial generational identities – as fathers, (great-)grandfathers and uncles. Considered in generational positions,[4] 7 were young fathers (aged 25 and under); 12 were mid-life fathers, most of whom were biologically related primary caregivers for children or stepfathers (and aged between 26 and 45); and 6 were kinship carers[5] (aged 38–73). One of these was an uncle who was in the process of securing state-recognised parental responsibility, and one was a great-grandfather who has secured a Special Guardianship Order already. One participant was a maternal grandfather and, although he was the most resourced and did not have significant family responsibilities, reflecting a more traditional and middle-class experience of grandfathering, he did describe a history of family poverty intimately connected with the localities where the more impoverished of the MPLC participants lived.

In researching the experiences of men in different generational positions, this book is distinctive in that it foregrounds men's caring practices and involvement across the lifecourse as a lens through which to examine both contextual processes and the subtle intersections of gender, class and generation, demonstrating how they play out in, and produce, diverse experiences of caregiving in contexts of material deprivation for men over time. The extended insights provided into the care responsibilities and everyday practices of men in different generational positions were also interpreted against a backdrop of austerity-driven welfare and policy reforms and 'late modernity', a period characterised by more rapid social change than in previous periods (Miller, 2010a; see also Chapter 3).

The men who participated in MPLC were predominantly white and all were heterosexual and living in low-income families and urban neighbourhoods in one Northern English city, reflecting the thematic orientation of the study. Only 18-year-old Adrian, who was recruited via a housing association, was from a minority ethnic background. This was the outcome of the recruitment strategy, which involved collaborating with professionals working in low-income urban areas experiencing multiple deprivation. It is therefore reflective of the character of the populations who reside there and of those individuals that organisations typically reach and support. It is worth noting here that there is a collective need, both for researchers and services that support and engage with men, to develop and refine methodologies for accessing and researching with individuals from diverse backgrounds, especially with regards to race and ethnicity (see also Brooks and Hodkinson, 2020). Despite their differing generational positions and identities, the men shared several characteristics, however, particularly in terms of economic status. Overall, these men were *present* in their children's lives rather than absent, but most were living economically precarious lives. Their participation as providers and caregivers was therefore transitory (Roy, 2004) and varied in intensity across the lifecourse and across the participant sample. They had inadequate incomes, often because of their primary responsibility for children, inadequate access to employment or reliance on part-time, low-paid or insecure work, limited access to affordable childcare, diminishing access to welfare support and some experience of debt.

While the participants were asked to state their monthly incomes on a participant information sheet, many were reticent to fill this in. They indicated that this was not because of feelings of inadequacy or shame but because, reflecting the dynamic character of poverty and deprivation, their financial situations were rapidly changing and dependent often on external agencies. Most were reliant on the social security system in some form, either via welfare payments (including pensions), Jobseeker's Allowance payments[6] and kinship care payments. Most described intermittent access to the labour market via low-paid, insecure work. They were also variably marginalised by their age, generational position, gender (in terms of being caregivers as men) and social class and according to their residence in multiply deprived communities and localities. Thus, in determining the theoretical relevance of their circumstances to the research, they were considered low-income in relation to several key factors linked to (usually a lack of) social and material capitals and family configurations that increased their financial vulnerability.

Life-journey interviews comprised the main method, conducted with 26 core participants (see Appendix 1) to elicit their family histories and biographies. The aim of the interviews was to develop understanding of the men's individual and family histories and the conditions and processes shaping their caring responsibilities over time. Specific attention was paid to their involvements in caregiving and nurturing as part of their generational and familial roles. The conversations were in-depth and covered a diverse range of themes, typically orientated around their family lives and relationships and the processes that had led them to the specific set of circumstances and care responsibilities that they were experiencing at the time of interview. They were also asked questions about services and support in their lives, including where support may have been needed but was not accessible. The interviews began with an opening question about their life history, which gave the participants an opportunity to convey their own experiences and views (Bertaux and Thompson, 1997), as well as insights about the life journeys they had experienced to reach the circumstances they found themselves in. The participants were acknowledged as informants on the various contexts shaping their lives and family relationships and were key sources in revealing what had happened in their lives so far; how and why they had the responsibilities they did; and their feelings and reactions (Bertaux and Thompson, 1997). Such an orientation supported the generation of both factual and interpretive information and generated dynamic and longitudinal perspectives of their experiences. This included accounts of their movements in and out employment and associated poverty, processes of relationship dissolution and change and the extent to which these pathways were contoured by the dynamic interactions of state, family and market.

The interviews with the core participants were complemented by a photovoice task that was used to visually capture men's everyday care practices and for a period of participant observation at a community centre in one low-income ward of the city where the study was conducted. The centre was often referred to by the MPLC project partners as a significant resource and space of care and compassion for the men who resided in the locality. The time spent at the community centre incorporated a method that I conceptualise as 'walking photovoice', conducted with regular attendees at the centre. In alignment with the principles of ethnography, this combination of methods produced rich, 'thick' descriptions of the processes and impacts of poverty and disadvantage on contemporary family life; of the challenges that local and familial poverty presented for these men in raising children under conditions of hardship; and of the material contexts shaping these men's family practices and experiences. Images produced via these methods are included in the empirical chapters where analytically relevant. For a variety of reasons, only five participants agreed to participate in the original photovoice activity (see Tarrant and Hughes, 2020 for further discussion), and of these five, four agreed to participate in follow-up interviews which generated a small subset of qualitative longitudinal data that captured change and continuity in the lives of these men. All of these data are complemented by insights from professionals working for services with a remit to support men with complex needs or requirements for family support (see Chapter 4).

Given the diversity and heterogeneity expressed by the participants about their personal and familial trajectories, circumstances and family arrangements, it is important to acknowledge that the accounts of these men should not be considered representative of men in low-income families and contexts more generally. A common characteristic across the cases, however, was that these men were considered disadvantaged in current policy contexts and in their relationship to the state because of their family responsibilities and identities. Given that the interviews were conducted between June 2015 and July 2017, they also reflect men's experiences of recent welfare reform policies linked to austerity. In particular, the sample was diverse in terms of family forms, aligning with findings from wider demographic studies (for example, Kemp et al, 2004) that show that low-income families are more likely to have non-traditional structures. This includes lone parents or parents in reconstituted families; parents living in households where no adult is in employment; households headed by a teenage parent; families that have a sick or disabled child, a child or children under five or multiple children. Across the sample, varying relationship status and caring arrangements were described. Most men occupied otherwise unconventional gendered care arrangements as primary caregivers for young children as lone fathers, as fathers with primary responsibility for children even though in couples, in families where someone was disabled or as kinship carers, either seeking or with confirmed legal guardianship. Three of the participants, namely those men accessing support at the community centre, had lost access to their children but still identified as fathers. The specificities of these caring arrangements and their implications for men's identities and lived experiences are examined in more detail in Chapter 5.

A new direction for debate and an overview of the book

This book elaborates a new, sociologically informed perspective of the care responsibilities and family participation of men living in low-income families and communities to interrogate overdrawn public claims that they are largely uncaring, irresponsible and absent from family contexts. It does so in a context where the veracity and dominance of the discourse on the absent father and adult male (Robb, 2019) obscures the varied and diverse ways in which men in different generational positions participate as family members and citizens while also responding to broader structural, familial and policy change. The findings and analyses presented provide a concerted challenge to the simplistic and stigmatising images that are commonly and often unproblematically perpetuated in the popular imagination to construct these men's experiences. As a distinct departure from the largely cultural analyses of representations of absent and present fathers that currently occupy academic research, insights are provided of men's care responsibilities across the lifecourse and over time in contexts of deprivation, revealing:

- how and when men participate in family life in low-income families at different stages of the lifecourse;
- how men describe and make sense of their family relationships;
- the impact of being (increasingly) financially constrained on their capabilities to care; and
- the effects of the changing policy context under the conditions of political austerity on these processes.

A range of iterative processes across key domains are examined in this book that shape the men's personal, family, community and work lives and identities. This includes their childhood experiences, school years and transitions from education to employment, their welfare and employment histories, becoming a parent/grandparent or carer and other care responsibilities and interdependencies beyond those for whom the men were primarily responsible. In some cases, the men reflected on processes of disconnection from family life and loss of access to children. Men's financial trajectories, their practices of financial provisioning and their evolving support needs, networks and resources, including those that are locally embedded, are also considered. Within these diverse trajectories it is possible to discern multiple processes. This includes both similar and diverse patterns of care and dependency across the lifecourse; men's gendered relations within complex configurations of kinship across generations; how and why men engage and disengage from family life across the lifecourse; and the impacts of vulnerability and marginalisation on these longer-term processes both within and across households. Insight was also gained about who or what has influenced the direction of their lives in the context of the relational and socioeconomic opportunities and constraints they have faced (for example, Neale, 2021). In examining these processes and often divergent trajectories, MPLC interprets the accounts and narratives of these men as active participants in family life.

The significance of their relations and dependencies with service providers across the health and social care landscape in the public and third sectors is also explored, demonstrating their vital role in determining men's capabilities to care and participate in family life. These findings support fresh interpretation of several themes with practical application for policy and practice, including insights into intergenerational chains of care and support from the perspectives of men in low-income families; questions of the longer-term resourcing of families; issues of work–life balance, social support and deprivation; and, finally, implications for the life chances, health and well-being of fathers and their families.

The concept of family participation is developed across the chapters of this book both to navigate and render visible the diverse ways men engage in and contribute to low-income family life across the lifecourse and to soften some of the problematic dichotomies that dominate discussions of fatherhood such as absence versus presence, culture versus conduct, good versus bad parenting and so on. While these languages can be useful and have their place, they are less so for the analyses developed in this study, which sought to uncover the diverse set of fathering practices, identities and caring responsibilities that men in different generational positions engage in in low-income families and over time. Underscored by the unique methodological focus on men in different generational positions, it becomes more possible to account for family processes and the dynamic patterning of family life that produces a variety of caring arrangements for men. Certainly, looking beyond the father generation empirically towards the vertical chains of generational relations and identities that constitute families makes it possible to observe men's practices and engagements within a much wider set of interdependencies both within and across households. These are often obscured in a policy context that tends to prioritise the financial contributions of the father generation over men's practical and emotional investments in caregiving more generally.

As context to the main findings of the MPLC study, the next two chapters of the book engage with current debates and discussions in relevant interdisciplinary fields. Chapters 2 and 3 develop the conceptual framework for the book and aim to situate the MPLC research in the context of existing knowledge and understanding of low-income fatherhoods so as to chart the changing landscapes of policy and family lives. Chapter 2 traces continuities and change over time in the cultures and conduct of low-income fatherhoods, examining the dynamic and shifting relationship between representations and evidence of lived experience. The theoretical and conceptual ideas that have underscored the historical development of oppositional categorisations of father involvement and absence are synthesised and traced, interrogating the extent to which these inherently contradictory discourses have been perpetuated and sustained within and across different historical and policy contexts.

Given the lack of empirical attention to low-income fatherhoods in the UK, and to develop a framework for a dynamic understanding of their family participation, the book draws on and integrates key bodies of interdisciplinary and feminist scholarship in Chapter 3. Particular attention is paid to dynamic theorisations of family change and evolving relationships and dependencies across the lifecourse; transformations and transitions in masculinities, as ostensibly captured through shifts towards caring masculinities; the complex intersections of masculinities, family care and the doing of kinship; and poverty as a dynamic, social and relational experience that is influenced by changing family processes and practices. These chapters are developed to situate and support a more critical examination of the current state of debate and to make a case for broadening the empirical terrain in relation to men's care responsibilities.

The second section of the book (comprising Chapters 4 to 7) is based on the qualitative findings generated, which, together, develop a dynamic and context-sensitive rendering of men's family participation in low-income contexts. It is important to note here that all reference within the data that makes participants identifiable is anonymised throughout these chapters in accordance with the overall ethical orientation of MPLC.

Chapter 4 develops discussion of the outcomes of interviews and a knowledge-exchange workshop held with professionals working for local services and the council who had a remit to support men with complex needs in the city. Their knowledge and understanding of the local and national policy contexts shaping the family lives and participation of low-income men in the city was elicited to develop an informed understanding of whether and how particular policy contexts influence men's abilities to fulfil their care responsibilities and relationships.

Chapters 5 and 6 comprise in-depth examinations of the narratives of the core MPLC participants (whose circumstances are described in more detail in Appendix 1 and throughout the empirical chapters). Interpretations of the biographical narratives generated are presented to produce rich insights into the social and relational dimensions of men's lives, as well as the hardships and constraints that impinge on their efforts towards their families. Chapter 5 begins by elaborating the diverse caring arrangements described by the men, as well as the dynamic processes and family trajectories of both the participants and their family members, which determined how their caring arrangements came to be. Providing extended evidence and insights like those presented at the start of this chapter, the cases and analyses presented here demonstrate further evidence of the clear disconnect between individualising public and policy representations of marginalised fathers and families living in poverty that construct them as absent, uncaring and partly responsible for the perpetual intergenerational transmission of poverty and deprivation. Instead, the wide range of emotional and material investments and interventions that are made by men in these contexts to sustain families are examined. Through conducting analyses within and across cases, the contexts of significant hardship through which men from different generational positions engage in a range of caring practices are also compared to reveal the especially pernicious and divergent intersections of difference that produce disadvantage for these fathers.

This is followed by consideration of men's familial economic circumstances and provisioning practices in Chapter 6. In this chapter, aspects of the financial and material constraint that impinge on men's efforts toward their children are explored as key processes. Also examined are how men's caring arrangements and narratives about their financial circumstances intersect, and how men engage in a range of everyday, but also future-orientated, strategies to sustain their families. These analyses are organised temporally, focusing on men's accounts of their everyday struggles and negotiations around finances, their vulnerability to external shocks, which have much longer-term consequences, and, finally, their anticipated economic futures.

Chapter 7 takes a different, but nonetheless theoretically relevant direction, focusing on the experiences of men residing in a low-income locality in the city where the MPLC study was conducted. This chapter reports on the ethnographic methods employed at a community centre in this locality that was observed as an important site of support, care and connectedness. In accessing some of the more marginalised men in the city, it was possible to observe how and why being a father or carer remains an important identity for men, even when access to children may have been compromised or lost. The limits to men's family participation are also considered via the lens of their local engagement, social networks and community participation. This chapter illustrates the deprivations of the contexts that shape men's identities, revealing the significance of the community centre as a key policy intervention for creating a space of collective engagement. This is especially valuable to the older men, for whom connections to family have become more tenuous. The main argument elaborated here is that an understanding of locality is integral to the development of a rich, multi-layered understanding of the contexts shaping men's participation in family life over time.

In Chapters 5 to 7 I present data alongside artistic plates developed with socially engaged artist Katie Smith, whom I met not long before the conclusion of the research. These are based on some of the empirical data from the study and were developed as a public engagement tool for an event at the University of Lincoln that was held in July 2018. We bonded immediately over a shared passion for tea and cake and the desire to think creatively about how we might work towards a more inclusive society by revealing, speaking directly to and challenging broader structures of inequality and power, using research findings. We decided to explore ways in which we could work together to produce creative outputs from MPLC. Katie thought that traditional letterpress prints would be the best medium for this work, not least because each design is completely unique and cannot be replicated, much like the narratives of the fathers in the research. Once the posters were designed, she worked closely with a Bristol-based organisation called the Small Print Company,[7] who printed them. Exemplars of these prints are interspersed with the photovoice images throughout the empirical chapters where analytically relevant.

The book concludes by connecting key strands of analysis advanced across each of the chapters. In Chapter 8 the key findings of MPLC are reiterated to draw conclusions about men's family participation in low-income family contexts. Considered are the extent to which men's dynamic histories of deprivation, caring arrangements, familial economic circumstances and connections to locality either mitigate against or intensify the challenges of care and provisioning for men in low-income families. The thesis of the book is also reclarified, namely that while policy and lay discussions of fathers in deprived contexts allocate blame to men for family absence, the narrow empirical focus on households and on the role of 'father' as a generational identity serves to obscure the variety of often vital ways in which men participate in family life at different times. Longitudinal and generational analyses reveal circumstances when the doing of family supersedes gender, such that men who are more resourced and capable of taking on care responsibilities do so, albeit where state support is lacking yet much needed. These arguments are elaborated throughout the book.

2

Low-income fatherhoods
in historical and political context

The extent to which men's relationships and lived experiences in low-income families and contexts have been addressed in academic debates and discussion is examined in this chapter. Superficial readings of interdisciplinary literatures that engage with questions of men, poverty and family and community life show that they make strong assertions that men's experiences are a key area of empirical neglect. Yet, these observations only serve to re-enforce, rather than address, their invisibility.

Drawing on an interdisciplinary scholarship from social history, sociology, social policy and social geography, the questions of how and why the social and relational dynamics and lived experiences of men in low-income families and contexts are often rendered invisible are interrogated. In-depth engagement with the literature explains the dominant and historically rooted policy preoccupation with fathers living in low-income families, which locates them within 'problem' and 'underclass' families, considers them absent, and relegates them to the margins of social and familial lives in the low-income localities and communities of urban Britain. This history has predominantly steered and underscored contemporary academic interest in the cultural politics of representational contexts and the sustained focus on crisis and father absence. While it is not possible to provide an exhaustive account of the histories and evolving policy contexts that have rendered empirical accounts of low-income fathers invisible in this chapter, tracing their development and intersections is vital to a more comprehensive understanding of men's family participation in low-income families over time.

Bridging these disciplines further serves to highlight the limitations of existing knowledge and understanding, as well as the fragmented and partial character of empirical focus on low-income men, their familial identities and the social, relational and temporal character of their family participation. Insightful pockets of research, ranging from classic urban community studies conducted in Britain to contemporary international contexts, are drawn together to situate the findings of the MPLC study within this broader historical, political and geographical terrain.

Concepts of absence and presence are also critiqued further, particularly in the context of discussions about fatherhood which define the current state of debate. A case is made in this chapter to bring evidence of the relational and social dimensions of men's lives in low-income contexts more fully into view.

Histories of low-income fatherhood: culture versus conduct

The exclusion of men in low-income contexts from academic research appears to be nothing new. It is in fact part of a broader historical process of stigmatisation in which working-class men and fathers are portrayed in ways that do not necessarily mesh with the realities of low-income family life. A notable body of social-historical research has begun to problematise persistent representations of working-class fathers as absent and disinterested in family life, via observation of ongoing discrepancies between the cultures and conduct or images and practices of fatherhood (LaRossa, 2012). This work suggests that public representations of fathers that pathologise families and conflate social and economic decline with the failings of individual fathers have always existed and have often obscured the empirical realities of these men's family lives.

An increasingly cohesive body of historical and archival research is questioning the extent of men's historical marginality from the home and family life more generally. In the three decades since 1990, social scientists researching in the Global North have been documenting what they consider to be an emerging cultural shift towards father involvement and engagement (Brooks and Hodkinson, 2020). Framed using the language of emerging or 'new' fatherhood (Dermott, 2003), father involvement is conceived as a distinctive shift from patterns established during industrialisation, where men were often considered to be marginal and even liminal family figures, and economic provisioning was considered a central pillar of male identity and good fatherhood. The contemporary language of 'new' fatherhood has been used to capture greater fluidity in models of fatherhood, and shifts in expectations that men are both nurturing and engaged with their children.

Yet the development of a more 'sophisticated historical knowledge of the family' and of masculinities throughout the 21st century (Arnold and Brady, 2011, cited by King, 2013) is challenging the recency and novelty of these more involved models of fatherhood by uncovering accounts of men's actual practices of caregiving over much longer time frames, including in low-income families and communities. Revealing the hidden practices and narratives of fathers of the past (for example, King, 2015; Robb, 2019), affectionate and 'family orientated' masculinities (King, 2013) are being found in evidence across numerous historical periods, in communities and places throughout Britain, and irrespective of social class (Davis and King, 2018).

Described as the pioneer of fatherhood research (Doucet, 2020), John Tosh was one of the first historians to focus on both the history of masculinities and the 'domestic' lives of men in middle-class families in the Victorian period (Tosh, 1996). Tosh categorises four different 'types' of fatherhood observed at this time that describe a spectrum of men's involvement in the physical and emotional aspects of parenting children. These include the absent, the tyrannical, the intimate and the distant father. At the extremes, the absent father is described as making infrequent interventions into the lives of his children, with rare involvement in the discipline or leadership required of men of this period. The harsh, tyrannical father is present and involved but practises violence to enforce his authority. Reflecting varying patterns of protection and provision for family regardless of social class, distant and intimate fathers express emotional involvement and affection but to varying degrees (Tosh, 1999). While this typology may appear static and to reify practices of fathering, Tosh acknowledges that these are not fixed positions and that they shifted for fathers, often in line with changes in their familial circumstances and across the lifecourse. Thus, a crucial contribution of his research is that fathers' roles and the extent of their involvement and time spent engaged in family life have always been fluid and diverse and have always fluctuated and evolved over time. In line with contemporary research, Tosh also identifies the significant role of industrial capitalism in marginalising fathers from domestic life, while at the same time reinforcing their role as providers and criminalising non-support and the desertion of families by so-called 'home-slackers' (Tosh, 1999: 230).

Social historian Laura King (2013, 2015) dates the shift towards men's greater involvement in family life to the interwar period, and indicates an intensified interest in fatherhood among the media and in individual families from the 1950s (Davis and King, 2018). Public interest at this time was connected to reconstructions of the family unit as self-sufficient and capable of meeting the varied needs of its members, as well as an ostensible shift towards democratisation in couple relationships (King, 2013). In developing a more sophisticated history of men and masculinities in the context of family life, King further illustrates the fluctuating prominence and visibility of fatherhoods in popular culture, which were sometimes celebrated and at other times demonised (King, 2013). While King's synthesis of historical evidence and research offers glimpses of family-orientated masculinities in working-class families across Britain, she argues that these stories remain largely untold (King, 2013). As Horsley et al (2020) observe, working-class and low-income families have seldom been the object of analysis, despite being subject to varying forms of governance over time. In historical research, where the experiences of men in low-income families have been examined, it remains the case that wage earning continues to be presented as the most valued father practice. Consideration therefore tends to be given to men's role as breadwinner rather than caregiver (Strange, 2012).

Important social historical interventions like those by King (2013, 2015) and Strange (2012) are now beginning to reveal evidence of men's emotional investments in their family and community lives, however. There are notable critiques, for example, of the ways that urban, working-class fathers' parenting skills have been historically portrayed and represented as disruptive and absent. In their classic ethnographic study of family and kinship in a working-class community in East London, Young and Wilmott (1978, pp. xii–xiv), describe the disconnect between portrayals of the manual workers who resided there, and their observations of their lived experiences. They state:

> manual workers are said to be shiftless, lazy, improvident, rascally, uncultured, acting for themselves alone. We could not, on the basis of what we found, subscribe to any such condemnation ... their poverty was accompanied by a sense of family, community and class solidarity. By a generosity towards others like themselves, by a wide range of attachments, by pride in themselves, their community, their country and by an overflowing vitality.

The archival research of historian Julie-Marie Strange also investigates what being, and having, a father meant to working-class families in the Victorian era and is doing important work to reintegrate and connect the paternal figure within the emotional worlds of their families, offering new relational accounts of their lives (Strange, 2012). Her research lends additional weight to the observations of Young and Wilmott and is revealing of empirical examples of father investments in family in an earlier period than that examined by King. While mindful not to overly romanticise the experiences and contributions of working-class fathers, she unveils the love, care and kindness demonstrated by many men in such contexts. Her exploration of Victorian working-class paternal identities and experiences also acknowledges the contrasts between their representation and their lived realities, as well as distinct discursive parallels between social portrayals of today's working-class fathers and their Victorian working-class counterparts. She notes that during the period of her study (1865–1914) working-class fathers were frequently portrayed as absent, feckless or 'rough, drunken and profane' (Strange, 2015: 1) and 'othered' just like today's fathers, often 'without interrogating what those experiences might be or, how working-class actors invested meaning in paternal identities or processes' (Strange, 2015: 3). Thus, the lived experiences, behaviours and attitudes of men in these contexts were continually misrepresented, demonised and rarely explored empirically. Like their working-class, female equivalents, Strange argues, these men have long been figures of class disgust and disdain (Tyler, 2008, cited by Strange, 2015). Social-historical research thus confirms that the paradox of fatherhood has a much longer history, warranting greater attention to the complex and evolving relationship between the images and realities of low-income fatherhoods today.

The hyper-visibility of low-income fathers in contemporary social policy and welfare contexts

It is to contemporary images and representations of low-income fatherhoods in popular and policy discourse that this chapter now (re)turns. Expanding on arguments established in Chapter 1 which initiated critique of debates about father absence in popular form, this section of the chapter elaborates social sciences debates in which low-income fathers have perhaps been most visible, albeit through attention to their discursive construction as absent. Indeed, while some social historical work is unsettling the historical separation of men from the home and family through the discovery and analysis of archived evidence, the current orientation of interdisciplinary analyses of policy and welfare contexts that are pertinent to low-income families means that empirical accounts from fathers have not routinely been used to inform debate.

As noted in the introductory chapter, the carefully crafted myth of a feckless and dead-beat underclass of absent fathers remains a continual component of contemporary policies and discourses that emphasise and prioritise the deficiencies of individuals in the causation of poverty. While both persistent and enduring, as Robb (2019) notes, the father-absence discourse experiences intermittent periods of resurgence in line with key historical moments and policy shifts, where it is reimagined with different emphases and inflections at different times. When traced alongside policy and welfare approaches to poverty and low-income family life, there is a clear pattern of overlap.

Key social and economic changes in industrialised economies that have produced a shift from industrial to post-industrial societies have been accompanied by continuity in policy focus on poverty and inequalities as conditions rather than processes (Lambert and Crossley, 2018). A dominant policy response to poverty over time has been to seek to remedy family failings and the perceived and stubborn 'tangle of pathology' (for example, Abdill, 2018) that is thought to characterise them. Premised on this framing, governments have observably pursued punitive policies rather than those that prioritise the provision of welfare (Welshman, 2013; Lambert and Crossley, 2018) to address these issues.

Scholars like Macnicol (1987), Welshman (2013) and Lambert and Crossley (2018) have traced the historical rise and decline of different labels for poor or 'problem' families over time, revealing a rich picture of continuity and change. Each a precursor to another and originating in the principles of the English Poor Laws, they begin with the 'residuum' of the 1880s, followed by the 'unemployable' of the 1900s, the 'problem family' of the 1950s, the 'underclass' of the 1980s and 1990s and, finally, the 'troubled families' of Broken Britain in the present day (cited by Lambert and Crossley, 2018). Despite linguistic change in the labels used to demarcate these families historically, Welshman (2013: 230, cited by Lambert and Crossley, 2018: 88) identifies commonalities in these periodic policy rediscoveries. This includes: 'ascribing undeservingness to sections of the poor; scapegoating and stereotyping their behaviour; similarities in the form and functions of labelling as a process; emergence during crisis or exposed through rising affluence; and the difficulty of applying such conceptions on practical policy and verifying their results'. While concepts of poverty have therefore changed under successive governments, the damaging effects of these constructions of low-income families persist.

The intensity of focus on absent fathers and an ostensible 'crisis of fatherlessness' has notably accompanied these cycles of rediscovery and has often been seized upon in explanations of a range of contemporary social problems. The intergenerational implications of absent fathers for young people can be traced back to the 1960s, in the context of a wider set of anxieties about the impacts of the long absences of men who had fought in the Second World War for child development and socialisation (Boothroyd and Perrett, 2008). Based on sex-role theory, it was assumed that boys who grew up with only a mother figure would develop a gender identity that was more feminised. It was not until the late 1960s and early 1970s, however, a period when Sir Keith Joseph promoted the idea that 'cycles of deprivation' in families are rooted in poor parenting (Welshman, 2012), that social policy and welfare concerns about fatherlessness and 'father absence' really came to the fore (Lamb, 2000). These policy emphases were accompanied by an intensified desire, in academic research at least, to quantify the extent of men's engagements in family life, cognisant with the dominance of the quantitative paradigm in fatherhood research and a methodological preference for time-use methodologies that measured the division of labour between mothers and fathers and time spent with children (Lamb, 2000). Father involvement at this time was therefore premised methodologically on 'an accounting ledger perspective' (Daly, 1996).

In the late 1980s and 1990s these methodologies were problematised as the role of fathers gained a new visibility in the context of a pivotal and historic policy change associated with the Children Act 1989. Encapsulating a shift in focus from fathers' rights to responsibilities (Fox Harding, 1991; Featherstone, 2009), the Act promoted the idea of the 'involved father' and demonstrated a growing consensus that fathers have positive contributions to make to families that transcend economic provision (see also Smart and Neale, 1999). Accordingly, a diverse set of constituencies turned their attention to the behaviours of men as fathers.

Taking a pessimistic view of family change and preceeding this policy change, New Right-influenced conservatives considered rising poverty rates to be symptomatic of an emerging social underclass, an idea imported by Charles Murray (1984) from the US. According to Murray, based on his thesis on welfare dependency and the cultural transmission of the underclass, lone-parent families were the cause of a host of social problems because of their inability to provide an adequate moral environment for children (see also Lees, 2008). Attention at this time began to shift to considerations of the role of the father (Daniels, 1998), providing a new 'arena for the rehearsal of concerns about boys and adult men' (Featherstone, 2003: 247). Riots in the north-east of England in the 1980s, for example, were blamed on the erosion of respectable working-class masculinities and linked to a decline in marriage and the rise of absent-father families (Featherstone, 2003). These discussions also consolidated the relationship between lone motherhood, absent fatherhood and long-term state and welfare dependency (Lister, 1996). Despite being the preserve of New Right commentary and thinking, the idea of father absence as a causal explanation for many of society's ills had purchase and was taken up by those with a variety of different political and theoretical perspectives (Williams, 1998). Ethical socialists Dennis and Erdos (1992), for example, linked the growth of fatherless families to increased crime in areas of the UK in the early 1990s. In their view, the family implicitly functions to make men 'useful' in society (Collier, 1998) and both the loss of a patriarchal family figure through the erosion of the breadwinner father and the demise of the family are seen to increase the criminality of young men. Dennis and Erdos did not accept, however, that these broader societal problems could be understood solely as the preserve of an inner-city underclass. Feminist Beatrix Campbell (1993) argued that lone-mother households and the absence of fathers were caused by differences in the ways men and women respond to their economic woes. Her analysis suggests that men adopt destructive practices and approaches while women seek strategies of survival rooted in social solidarity (cited by Featherstone, 2009, also see Williams, 1998).

The new 'Third Way' politics of the Labour government that was elected in 1997 were the precursor to the Conservative–Liberal Democrat coalition government that came to power in 2010. New Labour aimed to develop policies and politics designed to transcend 'New Right' and 'Old Left' policies, constitutive of a modernised social democracy that was committed to a flexible approach to ensuring social justice (Churchill, 2020). Over three terms of office, the social consequences of poor parenting became a major focus for policy and an array of interventions were subsequently developed (see Featherstone, 2013 for a detailed review). In relation to poverty, New Labour developed the langauge of 'social exclusion' (Lambert and Crossley, 2018), which, like other iterations before it, also eventually came to be recognised as a *condition* of the poor, rather than produced by broader socioeconomic *processes.* This thinking was foundational to the increasingly punitive welfare reforms introduced under the auspices of austerity that were to follow.

Austerity Britain: absent fathers, deprived localities

The 2008 global economic recession ruptured social policy debates (Churchill, 2020). In 2010, the Conservative–Liberal Democrat coalition government was formed while the UK economy was in recession (Ridge, 2013) and brought in an economic programme that aimed to reduce the national deficit and achieve economic stability.

As in other industrialised economies across the world, a political programme of austerity was implemented which comprised reforms that fundamentally reduced government spending and the size of the state (Ridge, 2013) in favour of the private market (Kitchen et al, 2011). The hitherto unprecedented cuts to social security provision and the retraction of the service sector, which predominantly employs women, had disproportionate effects and resulted in rising unemployment, deepening poverty and entrenched social inequalities (McKay et al, 2013; Ridge, 2013; Reynolds, 2020). As a population more likely to be in receipt of welfare and to rely on public services, women on low incomes and in minority ethnic communities endured the worst of government policy change in the ensuing years (MacLeavy, 2011; Jupp, 2017; Canton, 2018; Women's Budget Group, 2018; Hall, 2019). The decimation of state-supported services also placed additional pressures on families who were required to take on the greater share of the 'caring burden' (Power and Hall, 2017). Expectations placed on families were reinforced by neoliberal discourses of individualisation and self-responsibility, requiring citizens to take personal responsibility for the welfare of both themselves and others (Jensen and Tyler, 2012; van der Heijden et al, 2016). Representing a shift from what Wacquant (2010) describes as a Keynesian 'nanny state' to a more authoritarian 'daddy state', a punitive politics of welfare disgust and anti-welfare sentiment was crafted, underscoring a regime of tough welfare reform that had the aim of ending entitlement and worklessness (cited by Jensen and Tyler, 2012: 5).

Wrought by these wide-scale economic and political ruptures, the global economic recession and the associated episodes of civil unrest expressed through the 2011 urban riots across Britain that were discussed at the start of this book, were catalysts for a resurgence of moral claims about the existence of 'feral' parents and 'underclass' families, which came to be known as both 'troubled' and 'troubling' families in policy terms. Parents were categorised as deserving and undeserving, dependent on whether they were deemed to be engaging in 'good' or 'bad' parenting (Jensen and Tyler, 2012). The contemporary (re)discovery of fatherlessness has therefore been examined more recently as a key facet of the cultural politics of austerity and family life (for example, De Benedictis, 2012; Jensen and Tyler, 2015).

These debates demonstrate how the explanatory power of the discourse of absence became embedded in and enhanced by narratives of poor and 'feral' parenting, which were employed to account for what became framed as 'riots of the underclass' (De Benedictis, 2012; Tyler, 2013). Buttressed by well-rehearsed cultural framings of poverty and disadvantage in political and media arenas as being the product of personal failures, choices, morals and the genetic deficiencies of these families (Gillies, 2007; Tyler, 2013), government intervention was posited as the only route to encouraging these ostensibly fatherless, 'ineffectual' families back on track (Harker and Martin, 2012). Such framings were mobilised to contain the real meanings behind the discontent expressed at this time of significant civil unrest; to divert attention from wider structural, economic and political inequalities affected by encroaching neoliberal socioeconomic policies (see also Tyler and Jensen, 2012); and to lay the groundwork for wider public consent for shifting from protective and liberal forms of welfare to penal neoliberal 'workfare' regimes (Tyler, 2013).

A new set of imaginative and cultural representations of fathers failing to match up to the cultural imperative of involved and engaged fatherhood later came to be embodied in negative stereotypes of the welfare-dependent father (for example, De Benedictis, 2012; Jensen and Tyler, 2015). Public condemnation of welfare dependence accrued to particular kinds of families or 'national abjects', including the 'benefits broods' that featured heavily in 'poverty porn' TV shows like *Benefits Street* (Allen et al, 2014; Jensen, 2018; Shildrick, 2018), as well as single-mother households from which a feckless father is absent. Jensen and Tyler (2015) develop an insightful analysis of the framing of the case of Mike Philpott to evidence these processes. He was found guilty of the manslaughter of six of his children in 2013. The case was a pivotal moment in which the increasingly intensive focus on benefits broods in the media and popular culture became intertwined with narratives for legitimising welfare reform. Jensen and Tyler (2015) suggest that media emphasis on these *particular kinds* of failing, chaotic and dysfunctional families came to function as a 'technology of consent' for a much deeper programme of reform. Fears of a parent crisis were therefore used to justify the policing, discipline and blame of families thought to be morally deficient and socially responsible for their poverty, and have been used in social policy and popular discourse ever since to justify increasingly punitive state policies towards families (Jensen, 2018; see also De Benedictis, 2012).

While austerity politics have legitimised the intensification of neoliberal ideologies and policies around parents (Quaid, 2018) who are constructed as agents of both blame and change (Tyler and Jensen, 2012), the 2011 riots also became the latest in a long history of episodes of civil unrest and crisis in British history in which the figure of the troubled young, working-class male has been presented as the main symbol of disruption (Hebdige, 1988, cited by McDowell, 2002). It is, as McDowell (2014) notes, the activities and identities of these 'working-class rebels' that most interests the press and social scientists alike, often at the expense of scholarly attention to more 'ordinary' young men and fathers.

Located in this evolving historical and policy context, myths of fatherlessness today should therefore be recognised as situated within resurgent policy approaches to family and locality-based poverty that pathologise men and low-income families and problematically assume that the issues they experience are a product of their own personal failings, behaviours, choices and life-styles (Daly, 2018; MacDonald et al, 2020). Jensen (2018) cautions that when individual parents and families are castigated for their alleged moral failings, widening socioeconomic inequalities and the structural conditions in which families exist are also being overlooked. Structural inequalities like material disadvantage and lack of income are downplayed through the depiction of the family unit as the intergenerational transmitter of poor norms, values and practices (Gillies, 2007; Daly, 2018). An apt example of 'voodoo sociology', these are zombie arguments (MacDonald et al, 2014) that have been subject to considerable challenge and critique by sociological research, yet are resilient in their dominance and visibility in public discourse.

In the context of historical, policy and academic debate, fathers in low-income contexts are currently most visible in these cultural analyses of family lives and as figures of disdain within a wider politics of parent blame. Sociological attention has therefore predominantly been directed towards explanations for how representations and images of low-income fatherhood have come to be weaponised as part of an agenda for welfare and policy reform. Just as in the past, men's lived experiences of low-income family life subsequently remain largely out of view. In what follows, the relative (in)visibilities of men's experiences in low-income contexts are examined, identifying what might be gleaned from literatures that consider the structural processes contouring men's experiences and transitions across the lifecourse.

The (in)visibility of low-income fathers in social sciences research

Notwithstanding the relatively enduring and pervasive character of stigmatising accounts of low-income and working-class fathers in the dominant imagination, the contexts that form the backdrop against which men experience fatherhood and engage in family practices are undoubtedly changing. As policy and research interest in fathers has continued to gather momentum, only relatively few studies have focused empirically on men in low-income family contexts. Neither are there developed analyses attentive to social class (Braun et al, 2011) or the structural inequalities that produce different experiences of family and poverty for men in different places. Where low-income fathers are occasionally acknowledged or considered in academic research, the analytic lenses through which studies are conducted often mean that men's experiences from their own perspectives are often obscured from view. The perpetuation of negative notions of men in low-income contexts as *failing fathers* in policy terms is therefore reinforced not only by a limited and fragmented evidence base but also by the kinds of questions that are explored within different disciplinary sub-fields. Stigmatising labels of feckless and irresponsible men therefore deflect attention from questions about how societies might instead be *failing their fathers* (see Mincy et al, 2015) and by implication, their families.

Changes in the cultures and conduct of contemporary fatherhood must be understood in the context of the wider structural changes and the rapid socioeconomic transformations that characterise the early part of the 21st century. In a recent intervention on the evolving and intersectional relationship between masculinities and social class, Ward (2020) attributes the massive shifts that have been identified, in both economic and gendered relations, directly to processes of neoliberal governance and deindustrialisation. Alongside individualisation (discussed further in Chapter 3), these processes continually shape adult lifecourses over time (Pilcher et al, 2003). These macro-level processes have had uneven yet direct and distinct impacts on working-class communities, and have systematically reinforced class inequalities in ways that are often obscured in public debates which place emphasis on cultures of the poor. In an important call to action, Bottero (2008: 8) notes how many of the problems experienced by working-class communities today can be linked directly to longer-term shifts in the economic structure and political policy in Britain. She states:

> We should look at the impact of the closure of manufacturing industries which once dominated working-class communities; the neoliberal de-regulation of the labour market which has made their jobs less secure; the sponsoring of middle-class advantage through 'parental choice' of schools and the marketisation of education; the sell-off of council housing which concentrates in the most disadvantaged in the remaining estates; and the stalling of

incomes and expenditure at the bottom of the society whilst the wealth of the rich rockets.

Certainly, aspects of these processes were emergent in how the participants in the MPLC study narrated their family experiences. Since the 1980s, large-scale social and economic trends have produced ruptures, as well as continuities, in industrial communities and working-class life, linked to processes of deindustrialisation and the transition to a post-industrial economy (Ackers, 2017; Warren, 2017). These processes of decline, closure and the long-term ripple effect of deindustrialisation's aftermath and legacy have been a key area of interest in the social sciences. Much of the research about the impacts on men of Britain's evolving industrial history has focused either on the effects on their career histories or on the increasingly precarious and insecure transitions they have created for young, working-class boys entering adulthood (MacDonald, 1997). Additionally, while family sociologists remain concerned with theorising social change and the impacts of broader structural and societal changes on personal relationships (Gillies, 2003), the consequences of changes to the structure of education and employment for men in low-income families are often prioritised over change in their private and domestic lives.[1]

The implications of processes of economic change for working-class masculinities have been explored perhaps in most depth in research that examines the lifecourse transitions of young, working-class men living in localities marked by industrial decline and deprivation. At the intersection of gender, youth and education studies, this interdisciplinary body of research focuses empirically on the disproportionate effects these processes are having on the lifecourse transitions of young working-class men of the loss of well-paid, secure industrial and manufacturing jobs in many British towns and cities that relied on those industries (for example, Nayak, 2006; McDowell, 2014; Ward et al, 2017). These literatures make clear that labour market changes have led to greater insecurity and vulnerability and demonstrate how gender privileges derived from masculinity are undermined by age, class and occupation. Explanations of greater diversity in young men's transitions to adulthood have been established in rich bodies of empirical research. As well as the dominant focus on spaces of education (see Ward et al, 2017 for a full review), research has also examined young men's experiences of the streets, urban contexts and spaces of urban marginality (for example, Nayak, 2006; Wacquant, 2008a, 2008b; Gunter, 2010) and employment and workplaces (McDowell, 2003;

Roberts, 2013). Young fathers were an evident omission from these debates until very recently (for example, Neale et al, 2015).

Nevertheless, this extended and expansive body of research explores how encroaching neoliberal capitalism and governmentality, accompanied by the effects of employment change, are reshaping the lives and trajectories of working-class men not only in the UK but in post-industrial societies around the world (Walker and Roberts, 2018). Across international contexts, there is evidence that, regardless of educational attainment, many working-class young men today are growing up with limited opportunities for stable employment and are navigating increasingly risky life journeys. Young men living in the most deprived circumstances are coming to the age of work at a time when employment opportunities are increasingly scarce and the only work available is low paid and insecure. Evidence suggests that young men in low-income contexts are now less likely to move into professional occupations, since they lack the social and cultural attributes valued by such employers. They instead find employment in the lower-paid, casual service sector (Tarrant et al, 2015) with almost non-existent opportunities for progressive workplace transitions (Webster et al, 2004), or experience cycles of casual work with long periods of unemployment which confine them to an impoverished life-style.

Contemporary transitions to adulthood by young working-class men, who may also be fathers, therefore remain inextricably linked to locality, manual employment and changing gender relations and masculinities (Ward, 2015a; Ward et al, 2017). The increasingly visible problems of homelessness, poor mental health and suicide, and violence and substance abuse, have also been exacerbated by austerity and the associated programme of cuts to services, benefits and other forms of youth support (McDowell, 2017). MacDonald et al (2020: 12) conceptualise these issues as the outcome of 'a semi-permanent *constellation of external socio-economic pressures*' that have impacted on successive generations of families for decades. Declining job opportunities and cultures of worklessness alone therefore do not explain the persistent hardships experienced by deprived families and localities. Under austerity, a raft of heightened and extended pressures for families are also consequent on 'a contracting and disciplinary Welfare State, punitive criminal justice systems, poor-quality education and the physical decline of working-class neighbourhoods' (MacDonald et al, 2020: 27). Under these conditions, young men must now present themselves as either work-ready neoliberal subjects or 'individualised entrepreneurs', or, regardless of their existing dependents, care responsibilities or residence in towns where work for the less-skilled has all but vanished, become labelled as shirkers (McDowell, 2017). Reductions in welfare entitlements linked to austerity (Neale and Davies, 2015a) have further deepened these inequalities, shaping and intensifying young men's experiences of exclusion, marginalisation and the forging of ever more diverse and precarious trajectories to adulthood (Gunter and Watt, 2009). The recent work of social geographer Linda McDowell (2017) demonstrates how austerity policies have increased the vulnerabilities of young, working-class men and boys who, for the first time in several generations, have worse prospects for social mobility than their parents had.

MacDonald and Shildrick (2007) further suggest that, in their empirical focus on education, employment and training, 'mainstream' transitions literatures have failed to develop holistic analyses of young people's biographies of exclusion, which also incorporate leisure, drug using and criminal careers in the forging of alternative transitions (Maguire, 2020; see also MacDonald and Marsh, 2002; Webster et al, 2004).[2] Parenthood and family interdependencies, as key lifecourse domains, are underexplored aspects of the biographical career of young men. Debates in criminology and family policy indicate that young men who grow up in fatherless homes are particularly susceptible to becoming involved with gangs. Walklate (2007) suggests that this has been linked to their exposure to an impoverished social learning experience. Without fathers, it is thought that young men instead discover, and seek guidance about, their adult masculinity and male identity in the street. This means embracing a hegemonic masculine style in the deprived neighbourhood, conceptualised by Parsons (1954) as 'compensatory compulsory masculinity' (see also Chapter 7).

However, arguments such as these overemphasise their identities as tough, rough and uncaring and infer a complete separation from family. Roy's (2004) study of low-income fathers in the US suggests that local ecological processes such as gang involvement and police presence are not determining factors in whether men interact with family. However, local ecological processes are implicated in shaping men's more transitory participation in family life as providers and caregivers (Roy et al, 2004). More recent research with male youths from two poor and violent neighbourhoods in Medellin, Colombia also demonstrates that for young men who do not join gangs, families play an important role in helping them to develop a 'moral rejection' of crime and violence (Baird, 2012), as well as supporting them to carve out more positive transitions in adverse circumstances. Our own recent research (Ward et al, 2017) also illustrates the significant role of locality-based resources (including care-based relationships with support service staff) in influencing young men to create successful and 'safe' futures, empowering them and occasionally ameliorating some of their vulnerabilities. These place-based understandings of young men's identities offer an alternative to the wholly negative depictions of young, working-class men often captured by crisis discourses, revealing the importance of social and locality-based support structures in determining alternative lifecourse pathways. I contribute to the findings of this body of work further in Chapter 7, with a focus on the community centre as an important source and space of collective identity for men of all ages, including those who become disconnected from their families and identities as fathers.

Marginalisation processes and fathering practices

Returning to fatherhood debates, each of these structural and spatial processes is significant to the evolving relationship between economic power, poverty and father involvement and the challenges that this may present to low-income fathers or to men with caring responsibilities who experience unemployment (Shirani et al, 2012). Roy et al (2015) theorise these broad economic and political changes as marginalisation processes that impact on men's ability to establish themselves as good providers and family men. Indeed, masculinity is entwined with fatherhood ideals and being a good father and a breadwinner is foundational to how men achieve their status as men (Richards Solomon, 2017). In parallel with literatures concerning young, working-class boys' transitions, research about fatherhoods in low-income contexts demonstrates the significance of social context and place for family formation and the production of diverse experiences of fatherhood for low-income men across the lifecourse. Plantin et al (2003), for example, illustrate that men in low-income contexts are more likely than other fathers to experience more complex familial dynamics over time, including frequent critical transitions in and out of households, intimate relationships, father–child relationships and employment. As noted in the previous section, they may also face additional challenges linked to other ecological factors. These include the temptations of street life, gang activity, police presence, drugs and limited-opportunity structures. Despite these complexities, Plantin et al's research with low-income fathers suggests that living on a low income does not automatically equate to fathers' absence. They found that low-income men create strategies of resilience that enable them to overcome these barriers so that they continue to actively engage in caregiving for their children and the mothers of their children.

Undeniably, however, job instability and workplace inflexibility may produce a range of personal anxieties for working-class fathers, who may struggle to reconcile the norms of providing and caregiving and be fearful of being perceived as 'dead-beat' when unable to provide financially (Roy, 2004; Fox, 2009; Williams, 2010; Nomaguchi and Johnson, 2014; Roy et al, 2015). These processes are visible in men's discursive deployment of a 'domestic provision discourse' which, according to Willott and Griffin (1997), is characterised by feelings of emasculation, disempowerment, shame and inadequacy and associated with the perceived lack of ability to provide economically.

The diversity of these factors suggests that men's fathering practices often need to be 'responsive to changing circumstances and moments of rupture' (Meah and Jackson, 2016: 495). These findings also highlight the context and time-dependent nature of fathering practices. As Brannen and Nilsen (2006: 339; also cited by Meah and Jackson, 2016) observe, 'a father is always a father whatever his age … [and] fathering changes over the life course'. Poverty and social inequalities consequently impact in complex ways on men's family interdependencies and processes across the lifecourse in ways that warrant much further attention in the academic literature. In this book, findings are presented that demonstrate the intergenerational impacts and ripple effects of these processes across generations, either disconnecting men from their families or producing processes that require of men to step in and sustain their families.

While men's breadwinner identities are thought to be undergoing a process of destabilisation, more recent writings concerning fatherhoods in contexts of vulnerability offer a more optimistic view. Evidence generated with young fathers in a range of international contexts of social disadvantage (for example, Edin and Nelson, 2013; Enderstein and Boonzaier, 2015; Neale and Patrick, 2016) suggests that these young men are resistant to negative discourses of father absence, expressing a distinct desire to be involved in their children's lives while also fulfilling the prerogative to provide for them economically (see Neale and Davies, 2015a). Here, men's commitment to financial provision may be recast as a manifestation of familial commitment (Shirani et al, 2012). In this framing, alternative forms of care, such as the provision of financial advice to support younger family members, may be recast as practices of caregiving by men that disrupt otherwise feminised conceptualisations of care (see Hall, 2019). This involves framing the practices that may be obscured by narrower visions of care as part of the *work of family*. For Doucet (2020), attention to the complex entanglements of the concepts of breadwinning/providing and caregiving remains relatively underexplored but presents a potential opportunity to capture greater diversity in parenting practices. Developing an especially sensitive argument rooted in a feminist epistemology and mindful of the potentially negative consequences of reconceiving the concepts of breadwinning and caregiving, her reflections nevertheless indicate that there may be some value in moving beyond a binary conception and language of reconciliation. She acknowledges instead that breadwinning and caregiving weave together and, as such, breadwinning may be constructed as a key part *of* caregiving.

It is nevertheless significant that unemployment impacts on the abilities of low-income fathers to adhere to the broader cultural ethos of engaged fatherhood (Neale and Patrick, 2016). Edin and Nelson's (2013) ethnography of low-income fatherhood in Pennsylvania's Camden/Philadelphia metropolitan area demonstrates that if structural issues like unemployment, low wages and low skills persist, poor fathers can only continue 'to do the best they can' by their children and their families. As Eisenstadt and Oppenheim (2019) suggest, with a limited income it is much harder to be (at least perceived as) a 'good' parent, especially if lacking the resources required to ensure better outcomes for children.

Despite the potential to exclude some men from ideals of involved fatherhood, austerity and recessional processes are paradoxically thought to be intensifying the need for caregiving by men, underscoring the potential for alternative practices of family care to emerge. The economic recessionary processes of the last decade are therefore thought to be reconfiguring the care roles and responsibilities of men and women, as well as gendered relations and identities (McDowell, 2004). According to Boyer et al (2017), this is producing new gendered landscapes of care and a regendering of parenting practices. While feminist research about care work has predominantly focused on women, because they continue to be considered primarily responsible for unpaid care work and its organisation, recent research also indicates that men – especially fathers – are more likely to become involved in social reproduction during times of economic downturn (Henwood et al, 2010; Doucet, 2017).

A central question addressed here is how far male unemployment and redundancy may give rise to the renegotiation of domestic labour in households (see Boyer et al, 2017; Doucet, 2017). This is a contentious issue. In some circumstances, unemployment is thought to enable men to reconfigure their parental and personal identities (for example,

Smith, 2009). However, evidence that both predates and follows the economic recession suggests a mixed picture. In families where men are workless but nevertheless present in the household, a spectrum of engagement with children is apparent whereby fathers report either unusually high or low levels of engagement in developmental activities like reading, music and sports (Smith, 2009). According to Shows and Gerstel (2009), the extent of visibility of men's involvement is often linked to their employment status. Professional men are more likely to perform 'public fatherhood', involving more visible and observable forms of fathering, including attendance at public activities like sports and school events. Middle-class men may also engage discursively in public portrayals of involved fatherhood, despite working long hours and having the capital to buy in care that in various ways impact on how involved they really are as fathers. In contrast to their middle-class counterparts, working-class fathers have been found to be more intimately involved in their children's lives. These men tend to engage in practices of 'private fatherhood' (Gillies, 2009; Shows and Gerstel, 2009: Richards Solomon, 2017), which describes less publicly visible and heralded fathering practices, but more intense involvement in the day-to-day and hands-on care of children. Notably, fathering (and grandfathering, see Tarrant, 2013) is also performed in the public and private space that constitutes its caringspace (Bowlby et al, 2010; Meah and Jackson, 2016). The extent of men's involvement in low-income families may also be determined in part by the aspirations that fathers have for their children, as well as by opportunities shaped by the employment status of the mother of their children (Washbrook, 2007).

The practices of men in low-income families may therefore overlap with those of middle-class men, even though the context may be completely different. Comas d'Argemir and Soronellas (2019) suggest that this new gendered landscape affords low-income fathers with opportunities to invest more in caregiving and to assume primary responsibility for care. Their research finds that men are becoming new agents in care, linked to the wider social and cultural changes that influence how care is allocated.

However, research by Willott and Griffin (1997) questions whether there is a spatial convergence between men, the domestic sphere and their increased engagement in domestic roles when men's employment is disrupted. They argue that a simple occupation of the home space is not always indicative of progress towards more egalitarian attitudes toward caregiving and engagement in family roles (Miller, 2010b). For these researchers, unemployment and more time spent at home does not represent enough of a shift to confirm change in masculinities. For example, when fathers are present at home, this does not always result in positive outcomes for family dynamics. Dicks et al (1998) illustrate the negative relational effects that men's redundancy can have for family dynamics, including for women and children. Based on research with health, welfare and education service providers for families and communities affected by labour market restructuring resulting from coalmine closures in Wales, Dicks et al found that women experienced a great deal of anxiety and stress about the impact of the increased hardship on the family budget, especially because they were largely responsible for family purchases like food. They were also reportedly at the 'sharp end' of their partners' stress relating to their redundancy and worklessness, and often felt responsible for their partners' well-being. The presence of men in the home was also considered to be problematic for children. Child-rearing practices were affected, blurring the distinction between 'parent-as-authority' and 'parent-as-carer'. Paradoxically, men's authority, which had been derived from their daily absence, was eroded. Traditional divisions of labour and gender relations in such contexts were therefore perceived as 'ideal'.

These diverse findings suggest that, despite some optimism that regendering processes can 'undo' gendered binaries by shifting parenting practices within the private sphere (Boyer et al, 2017), there may also be unanticipated and invisible intra-household impacts within family contexts. Furthermore, as Boyer et al (2017) observe, the regendering of care may be more difficult to achieve in contexts where welfare and policy systems support only *some* men to be more involved in caregiving. Each of these arguments demonstrates the significance of unpicking what fathers say they do versus what they actually do.

Men and contemporary family poverty

The final section of this chapter turns to debates in poverty studies and the family poverty sub-field, where, as noted in Chapter 1, the social and relational dimensions of men's experiences of poverty have been identified as an area of absence and a future avenue for research (Ridge, 2009). Despite the powerful mobilisation of discourses about men as 'feckless' and absent and the pervasiveness of such narratives over time, particularly during times of crisis, understandings of men's experiences within families living in poverty, not just as fathers but as part of wider household and non-household interdependencies, remain underexplored and under-researched (Bennett and Daly, 2014; Ridge, 2009). A rare exception is Lisa McKenzie's ethnographic research on low-income families living on the St Ann's estate in Nottingham, where she specifically sought to uncover the accounts of 'missing men' (McKenzie, 2010). While the men she interviewed had strong friendships and family ties, she found that men, the sons, brothers and the 'baby daddies', did not participate in family life in the same ways as the women on the estate. They had very transitory lives and identities, and she notes that when she interviewed women on the estate, either in their homes or in the community centre, men were either leaving, on their way out or passing by. As an exemplar of the significance of research methodology for uncovering men's presence in low-income families, McKenzie instead sought to identify *their* spaces on the estate, namely where they were present, like the boxing gym, the barbershop and the flats where they hung out to play X-Box.

More generally, the empirical emphasis on women's experiences in poverty research is for good reason. The female-centred empirical basis of poverty research has proven necessary, given the gendered nature of poverty processes. Women are typically at a higher risk of living and remaining in poverty across the lifecourse (Bennett and Daly, 2014) and more likely to face specific challenges in achieving financial security both for themselves and for their families (Ridge and Millar, 2008; Ridge, 2009). However, narrow focus in poverty research on the household as a unit of analysis precludes wider analysis of resource and income distributions within family settings (Daly, 2018; Dermott, 2016), as well as gendered and generational interdependencies and family processes across households. Bennett and Daly (2014: 7) suggest that this methodological approach has the effect of conflating 'the effects of living arrangements on poverty with those of gender'. Inevitably, women's accounts of poverty, including as mothers, are not an exclusive story. As Ruxton (2002) argues, there is also value in interrogating masculinities and the specifics of male experiences of poverty as gendered. The relational experiences of poverty are also significant to men, not least for non-resident fathers. This group of fathers are more likely to be parenting across households and doing so in contexts of poverty and disadvantage (Dermott, 2016; Poole et al, 2016). There is also a paucity of attention in existing fatherhood research to the experiences of fathers who parent alone, who live separately from their children or who see them part time (Gatrell et al, 2015; Burgess and Davies, 2017).

Life in the UK is said to have become increasingly insecure and impoverished for many men (Ruxton, 2002). Indeed, an examination of poverty trends in the UK since 2012 confirms a trend of increasing insecurity for men (Dermott and Pantasiz, 2014), highlighting that gender disparities linked to poverty among men and women are less stark than they have been in the past. In fact, since the 2008 recession, poverty rates between men and women are converging (Dermott and Pantasiz, 2014). Linked to specific household and family circumstances, there are emerging groups of men experiencing poverty whose subjective experiences are rarely considered. This includes non-resident fathers and those who are solo living (Dermott, 2016; Dermott and Pantasiz, 2014). Reflecting a theoretical interest in the structural relationship between family and poverty (Daly, 2018), this research identifies men whose family configurations as single, childless men or as men resourcing children across households renders them more vulnerable to poverty. The impacts and risks of paying child maintenance for non-resident parents (who are usually fathers) are not fully understood, not to mention what happens when men enter new partnerships with others who also have care responsibilities. Dermott (2016) also notes that questions of poverty and disadvantage have not been central to research on non-residential fatherhood either, which has instead focused either on the impacts of absent fatherhood on child well-being or on debates about the rights and responsibilities of men in relation to contact and financial support. However, her analysis of the 2012 Poverty and Social Exclusion Survey reveals that non-resident fathers are more likely to have worse outcomes than resident-only fathers across all measures of poverty, deprivation and economising.

Poverty also has complex and sometimes differing implications for men and women (for example, Fodor, 2006; Strier et al, 2015). Fodor's research with couples in low-income households in Hungary exemplifies these differences, suggesting that men are more likely to experience 'gender role crisis' when they are too poor to fulfil expectations as a successful breadwinner. Couples in Fodor's study were identified as working to devise strategies to alleviate men's 'gender shame'. This included delegating the management of public shame to women; men's denial and 'learned ignorance' of finances and budgets; men's dominance in other everyday household matters; and the depiction of men as generous yet ignorant about money matters. From this perspective, poverty represents exclusion from the privileges of the dominant gender status, as well as economic hardship for men (see also Strier 2014; Strier et al, 2014). Aligning with evidence generated by the MPLC study, Bennett and Daly (2014) confirm that men are also more likely to express shame associated with being unable to provide financially and needing to rely on others and/or on benefits.

Several qualitative studies about intra-household and couple experiences of poverty also demonstrate gendered patterns of disadvantage in relation to budgeting and money management in low-income families, whereby women often bear the burden of restricted incomes (for example, Goode, 2010). Goode's study of men and household debt found that lack of job stability, reliance on benefits for substantial periods and/or addictions were important triggers of problematic debt for men. Responses to debt also impacted heavily on patterns of control and income management, and thus on couple relationships and dynamics. Women, who were often left with little access to money, carried an unequal burden of worry, while men were seen to control and manage finances often via internet and telephone banking (Goode and Waring, 2011). This research also suggests that male pride acts as a barrier to seeking advice around finance-related matters (Goode, 2012), although positive experiences of seeking help also helped to reinforce help-seeking behaviours (Goode and Waring, 2011). Neither Fodor (2006) nor Goode (2011) explores the intergenerational impacts of indebtedness and deprivation on wider family relationships – for example, impacts on men's relations with and responsibilities for children. Research in this area tends to consider the relational impacts of women's poverty on their children (Ridge, 2013).

Finally, Bennett and Daly's (2014) review of research examining the relationship between gender and poverty illustrates how gender acts as a key mediating influence on routes in and out of poverty, across the lifecourse. They develop a conceptual framework that features the family, labour market and welfare state, which, they argue, combine and interact to influence poverty incidence and experience. As an exemplar, they review the research of Demey et al (2013), who highlight the poverty pathways of middle-aged men living alone in Britain. The retrospective life histories they conducted suggested that unemployed men were more likely to have delayed family formation and thus appeared to be more disadvantaged than women, as indicated by their low socioeconomic status and lack of family resources. Bennett and Daly (2014) conclude that the investigation of lifecourse trajectories and increased use of methods informed by QLR would support an interrogation of the combined impacts of family, labour market and welfare state provisions, both on individual lives and on their links with poverty for men and women.

Concluding remarks

In this chapter questions of the extent of men's absence and presence in current interdisciplinary academic literatures have been interrogated, with specific focus on the dynamic relationship between the cultures and conduct of fathers in low-income families and localities. In tracing the history of these debates through contemporary social-historical research as context to contemporary representations of low-income family life, an argument about how and why men's family experiences have been absented, albeit perhaps inadvertently, has been carved. These observations reflect a clear rationale for bringing men's qualitative accounts of their family participation in low-income contexts back into view. While there are pockets of insightful research across these diverse disciplinary fields, the overall paucity of research evidence serves to reinforce the impression that men lack connectedness and relational identities in these contexts and that they are absent and, at worst, feckless and uncaring. The ongoing preoccupation with deficit, blame and disgust in policy and media arenas, alongside limited academic attention to men's qualitative and subjective experiences of family from their perspectives, therefore continues to render invisible the capabilities and contributions of men in low-income contexts, intensifying the absenting of evidence generated with low-income fathers and male caregivers in different generational positions.

3

Theorising men's participation in low-income families

This chapter develops the conceptual framework for the empirical chapters of the book, outlining how dynamic and temporally orientated constructions of the key themes, namely fathering, poverty and family, underscore a sociological conceptualisation and explanation of men's family participation in low-income families. Given the dearth of empirical attention to men's care responsibilities and the patterning of their family lives and participation over time in low-income contexts, it is important to elaborate these key theoretical starting points. The concept of family participation is foregrounded in this book to capture, but also widen the scope of, current academic and policy interest in the father generation and to better understand how, why and when men participate in low-income family contexts. Greater family diversity and increased opportunities for men to engage in family care over the lifecourse are linked to both structural and cultural changes and indicate the need to incorporate and account for the active family participation of other male carers, as well as fathers.

Four currently disparate yet interrelated bodies of knowledge are woven together, synthesised and considered in relation to low-income fathering. These are family diversity and dynamics; masculinities 'in transition'; the doing of kinship and family care; and approaches to theorising low-income family life. Drawing predominantly on feminist interdisciplinary literatures, the intersections of the gendered, classed and generational power relations that shape family relationships and structures are considered as foundational to the analyses and interpretations presented.

The chapter begins with a brief overview of qualitative longitudinal research as the key theoretical paradigm in which the study findings and conceptualisation of family participation are situated.

Qualitative longitudinal research: thinking dynamically

Given its intimate connection to the Timescapes programme of research (see Chapter 1), MPLC drew on perspectives and concepts from QLR. Taking the lifecourse as the central organising framework, QLR prioritises the temporal dimensions of lived experience to grasp the nature of social change (Neale, 2019). Research in this tradition demonstrates a commitment to an examination of how and why change is created, lived and experienced by individuals and understood by them in the context of broader societal shifts (Holland and Edwards, 2014). Referencing Hockey and James (1993), Hopkins and Pain (2007: 5) note that individuals live dynamic and varied lifecourses that are better envisaged 'less as the mechanical turning of a wheel and more as the unpredictable flow of a river'. A key aim of QLR therefore is to discern the unpredictable flows, turning points, transitions and changes that characterise lives as they unfold (Neale, 2021). More recently, QLR has also supported new substantive understandings of social change and continuities in the field of men and masculinities (Brannen and Nilsen, 2006; Bjørnholt, 2014) and in the development of fatherhood and fatherly identities (Miller, 2010a, 2018b; Shirani et al, 2012; Neale et al, 2015; Brooks and Hodkinson, 2020).

Lifecourse perspectives, which also have their origins in biographical approaches, have essential value for understanding changing practices in people's lives and the lived experiences of individuals and groups in the context of wider socio-historical processes. As Nilsen and Brannen (2014) note, such a perspective means that lives can be understood both over time and in particular times and places. Four interdependent ideas are brought together here to examine this intersectional relationship between biography and history (Mills, 1959; Elder, 1994, cited by Gray et al, 2016). These are that the historical periods in which people are born influence both what constrains them as well as what is available to them; that different life stages, like childhood, adulthood, old age and so on are socially constructed; that lives are linked interdependently, are relational and tied into kinship and social networks; and finally, that people have human agency which influences how they act in relation to others (Gray et al, 2016), thus acknowledging their strengths and capacities for change.

Building on these foundational ideas, the theoretical framework for MPLC and the analyses presented in this book are further premised on three additional components that aid in articulating a relational, context-specific and longitudinal understanding of men's family participation in low-income contexts and their adaptations to evolving social and material conditions.[1] These are:

1. that contemporary family biographies and lifecourses are characteristically complex and diverse;
2. lives remain linked and interdependent over the lifecourse, regardless of socioeconomic status; and,
3. social and policy contexts matter, especially when families are vulnerable or are at risk of vulnerability.

Pertinent to this interpretive and processual framework of family participation are the connections and articulations of men's individual lives and biographies with complex structural conditions and processes, including welfare and labour systems and a range of unequal power relations including gender, as well as class, age and generation. The concept of intersectionality is a valuable explanatory tool here for enabling a more nuanced understanding of gender differences as mediated and transformed by other categories of disadvantage. Rooted in the essential work of black and anti-racist feminist academics and activists (for example, Crenshaw, 1989; Brah and Phoenix, 2004; see also Hopkins, 2019), its use has burgeoned to support relational thinking about the diversity of individual lifecourses as they unfold, while also drawing attention to how mutually constitutive forms of oppression both intersect and interact in everyday lives. Intersectionality captures how social identity categories produce experiences of privilege and marginalisation and draws attention to the differences that exist *among* groups, as well as *between* them (Smooth, 2013). Analyses that explore the relationship between masculinities and intersectionality are rare, in part because the concept has been applied almost exclusively within a feminist framework in which men are considered 'other' because they are in possession of power and privilege (Milligan and Morbey, 2016). However, the diversity and contested character of masculinities that manifest through normative hierarchies, stratifications and exclusions that shift and change over time and space (Milligan and Morbey, 2016) means that there is value in thinking about intersectionality in the context of men's family participation across the lifecourse, in low-income family contexts and in the context of debates that examine the gendering of care.

These perspectives on the lifecourse and intersectionality undergird the overall framework of the book and are developed to support a more comprehensive understanding of men's family participation in low-income contexts as dynamic and diverse phenomena.

Families, caring masculinities and low-income life: a conceptual framework

The empirical neglect of men's lived experiences of family life as derived from their own perspectives means that the findings presented in this book necessarily need to be positioned within a broad interdisciplinary body of work. The previous chapter has gone some way towards situating the research and its findings in historical and political context and illustrated how evolving historical processes have exerted influence on, and reflect ideas about, men's family lives in low-income contexts over time.

The task of providing a comprehensive account of men's family participation in low-income contexts in the contemporary context is not straightforward. Relevant conceptualisations of family, masculinities and poverty are interrelated, highly complex in their own right and evolving over time as theoretical languages and tools become increasingly sophisticated. The empirical variety and diversity characterising men's caring arrangements, as well as individual variations in experiences of caregiving across the lifecourse as individuals adapt and change in relation to the care needs of other family members further adds to this complexity. In the remainder of this chapter more recent developments in scholarship examining family diversity, men and masculinities, and kinship and low-income family life are critically appraised and elaborated to develop and articulate the theoretical basis for men's family participation.

Family dynamics, diversity and social change

Families are an important lens through which sociological analyses of social continuities and change are observed and developed (Gillies, 2003; Naldini et al, 2018). A raft of sociological research demonstrates how family forms across European societies have shifted from extended to nuclear households, driven by the rapid processes of industrialisation and urbanisation that characterised the early 19th century (Gillies, 2003; Chambers, 2012). It was during this epoch that the breadwinner model of fatherhood first came to the fore (Williams, 2009). Amongst mid-20th century sociologists, the nuclear family, predicated on a distinct gendered division of labour between men and women, was often taken for granted (Williams, 2009; Gray et al, 2016). A much wider variety of household and family arrangements are more commonplace today, a period that has been described as 'late' or 'liquid modernity' (Bauman, 2000). Family patterns across Europe have undergone extensive transformations since the early 1970s linked both to changing economic pressures and to policy change. Towards the end of the 1960s increasing family diversity ushered in the end of the 'Golden Age of the Family' (Oláh et al, 2018), which constituted relatively stable marriage and birth rates, low divorce rates and a high prevalence of nuclear family forms. Greater diversity in family forms was driven by new opportunities for divorce and family dissolution, the postponement of marriage and parenthood (producing more prolonged transitions to adulthood) and the emergence of new forms of couple relationship (Oláh et al, 2018). Globalisation and economic restructuring (see Chapter 2) also resulted in the expansion of the service sector and increasing employment opportunities for women, while deindustrialisation and rising male unemployment have made women's paid employment and dual breadwinning more necessary (Dermott, 2008; Lees, 2008).

Associated changes in societal and family norms and in economic and legislative contexts have consequently produced more diverse family biographies and the destandardisation of family lifecourses (Oláh et al, 2018). This is most evident when contrasting the different lifecourse trajectories that men and women are likely to experience in relation to both the family and employment domains. Lifecourse research suggests that where men's lifecourse trajectories were once more stable and rigidly structured than women's, with fewer discontinuities, men and women's lifecourse trajectories have now started to converge and have become similarly irregular (Hutchison, 2019). Women's trajectories were once more tightly interwoven with the family domain, for example, which operates on nonlinear time and produces greater irregularities for women (Setftersten and Lovegreen, 1998, cited by Hutchison, 2019). Evidence indicates that the convergence of trajectories between men and women is linked most strongly to women's increased engagement in schooling and employment, while recent declines in employment stability have also led to much greater divergence and discontinuity in the lifecourse trajectories of men. Social class differences are also pertinent for producing differences in the lifecourse trajectories of young people, with implications for outcomes in adulthood. Less-affluent young people, for example, are more likely to enter into marriage, parenting and employment much earlier in the lifecourse than their more affluent counterparts (Hutchison, 2019).

New partnership and childbearing trends have also created greater diversity in family forms, including individuals and couples who remain childless, either through the voluntary or involuntary postponement of parenthood (for example, Dykstra and Hagestad, 2007; Hadley and Hanley, 2011); living-apart-together arrangements, where couples do not reside in the same household (Holmes, 2006; Duncan and Phillips, 2010); and an increase in single-parent families (often because of separation or divorce) and step- or blended families. The increased plurality of family forms has also led to greater diversity in fathering, whereby fathers now constitute a diverse group of individuals parenting in a wider range of circumstances (Lee, 2008). Varied family arrangements and trajectories are also reflected in diversities relating to sexuality and ethnicity, reflective of the increased prevalence and acknowledgement of same-sex families and diverse patterning and partnerships among migrants (Oláh et al, 2018). It is worth noting here that, while indicators like these are often interpreted as evidence of rapid social change, some caution against their ostensible speed and novelty (Naldini et al, 2018). Naldini et al (2018) note, for example, that renovation in family structures and practices has always been continuous and in line with broader societal change.

Questions of social change occupy a central place in contemporary theorising about the family and community life (Gillies and Edwards, 2005; Charles and Crow, 2012) and are highly contested. Gillies and Edwards (2005) develop a detailed overview of the two main theoretical perspectives that dominate public discussion and academic debate, before identifying a third. They argue that debates in the main are structured around the premise that social and economic changes profoundly influence how people relate in intimate and family life. The contexts for investigating family life are predominantly theorised in pessimistic view as being about demise, and in optimistic view as about transformation or as about continuity (Gillies and Edwards, 2005).

In pessimistic perspective, post-industrialisation is viewed as causing the detraditionalisation and individualisation of social life. The breakdown of ties, disintegration of moral frameworks and decline in values of duty and responsibility are perceived to place strain on families, undermine good parenting and damage social cohesion (Gillies and Edwards, 2005). The views of Murray (1984) and of Dennis and Erdos (1992) that were reviewed in Chapter 2 align with such perspectives, contending that both 'the family' and fathers with no useful familial role are in crisis in a way that has severe societal consequences.

The more optimistic view of social change is that greater diversity and the plurality of life-styles have generated new opportunities for choice and agency. In this perspective, opportunities for more fulfilling family and community relationships are premised on egalitarian values of respect and negotiation instead of duty and obligation. Individualisation theorists like Beck and Beck-Gernsheim (1995; 2002) and Giddens

(1991) contend that these changes have produced greater freedoms of choice, leading to an increase in equality between the sexes and the democratisation of family relations. Furthermore, fathers are afforded greater choice to reformulate their roles and increase their involvement with children (Lees, 2008). As Hollway (2006) argues, however, the complex processes of social transformation that produce individuals with capacities for autonomy, self-reflection and freedom of choice obscure considerations of their affiliations and care obligations. These are traditionally rooted in kinship and unequal power relations and require women in particular to put the care of others ahead of their own freedom of choice (Hollway, 2006).

A 'plus ça change' perspective has subsequently emerged that criticises individualisation theorists for their regeneration perspectives and 'pessimists' for their focus on demise in family and community lives (Crow, 2002; Gillies and Edwards, 2005). This perspective questions the extent of social change, highlighting the continued importance that is placed on family relationships and obligations by individuals, alongside the ongoing reproduction of privilege and inequalities within family contexts (for example, Jamieson 1998; Ribbens McCarthy et al, 2003; Edwards and Gillies, 2012). The extent to which family diversity and plurality in family forms can be considered new has also been questioned, especially as parenting continues to be a profoundly female activity and change has also been uneven and variable (Williams, 2004; Lees, 2008).

As wider socio-historical processes inevitably exert change on families, sociologists have increasingly turned their attention away from the macro approaches adopted by individualisation theorists and pessimists and have instead turned to inductive approaches that involve the theorisation of their 'inner worlds' (Daly and Kelly, 2015). Exploration of the complex sets of dependencies and interdependencies that constitute families as they evolve over time lends itself to a dynamic, processual perspective of family life, relationships and kinship obligations (Neale, 2000). Developing a theory of *family dynamics*, Bren Neale (2000: 1) suggests that 'the' family, as an ahistorical and essential institution has never existed. What do exist, she argues, and always have historically, 'are fluid webs of relationships and practices through which we define our personal, familial and kinship obligation. This fluidity operates not only historically, in terms of wider processes of change, but biographically, within the life course of individuals'. The family dynamics perspective not only destabilises 'the' family as a noun but explicitly captures how lives are lived relationally as well as in socio-historic context.

More recent sociological and feminist analyses of family have also sought to capture and explain the presence of power relations and inequalities that characterise family and household interactions. In this perspective, families are constructed as complex, multi-layered and diverse, and increasingly sophisticated theoretical tools have emerged for this purpose. The now late David Morgan's (1996; 2011) oft-cited and applied concept of family practices, for example, theorises families as spaces of performance, agency and negotiation (Daly, 2018). Rather than defining families as fixed or relatively static structures, family practices construct family as a verb, as something that is *done* and that we do and achieve. Here, the complex nature of family life is captured, including the diverse ways that roles and relationships are organised and enacted in everyday life. This includes anything from the sharing of resources to caring, meeting responsibilities and fulfilling obligations (Silva and Smart, 1997).

The interplay of personal biographies and social histories and the linking of history and biography are also intrinsic to a family-practices approach. Family practices are enacted, to some extent, in the context of predetermined or prevalidated structures (personal, legal and cultural) that influence but do not necessarily determine personal experience (see also Earley, 2017). Gatrell et al (2015) also point to the significance of a relational approach to families that acknowledges them as collective units in which lives are conceived as linked and lifecourse trajectories are configured variably over time by a myriad of individual ties, relations, obligations and exchanges with significant others, including partners, parents and children (see also Elder and Giele, 2009; Bedston et al, 2019). Moreover, the lifecourse perspective lends itself particularly well to 'an understanding of families as fluid, adaptable and with changing needs, depending on the status of the adult relationships and the ages and health of the children' (Gatrell et al, 2015: 226). In this formulation, family practices also aid in distinguishing broad conceptual languages in research about fathers. Morgan (1996) elaborates the distinctions between 'fathers' as individuals who have either biological or social roles; 'fatherhood', which describes discourses and representations; and 'fathering', which refers to social practices.

The family practices perspective has rarely been applied in contexts of poverty or low income, although Daly and Kelly's (2015) study of low-income families in Ireland is a notable exception and is discussed in more depth later in this chapter. They advocate for greater scrutiny of families as sites of power struggle, constituting processes and practices that actualise relationships and inequalities of class, gender and generation. Their work encourages an exploration of low-income family lives as situated within a wider set of kinship ties and interdependencies and 'as an arrangement of personal life' (also see Smart, 2007). Crucially for the MPLC study, this approach involves shifting focus away from the more functional arrangement of the household. These theoretical suppositions are taken up and applied in this book to develop a dynamic understanding of the internal family lives described by the research participants and the processes shaping their family participation over time and across the lifecourse.

Changing gender relations

Despite consensus about the increasing prevalence of diversity and change in family forms in the latter half of the 20th and early 21st centuries, there is much less agreement about the extent to which these demographic shifts have resulted in changes in gender relations, identities and practices, especially within family contexts. Nevertheless, as the discussions in Chapters 1 and 2 reflect, there are considerable and profound public anxieties about the implications of changes in gender relations in contemporary societies. Indicative of varying degrees of pessimism and optimism, the movement away from prescribed gender, sexual and work roles for men and women has long been at the centre of debate, social theory and anxiety (Williams, 1998). While wider demographic, economic, social and cultural changes have evidently impacted on family configurations and relations, the extent of change in gendered divisions of employment and unpaid family labour has endured as the central concern of these discussions.

Recent advances in the study of men in families are dominated by attention to the caring practices of the father generation, driven by evidence of men's greater participation in the lives of their children and recognition that fathering experiences have become more dynamic and complex over time (Roy, 2006). This is in part explained by the contemporary context in which men now come to fatherhood; a much more fluid context than previous times and one offering new possibilities (Miller, 2010a). A major strand of debate regarding shifts in men's roles and identities in family life focuses on the extent to which macro-level processes and socio-historical processes, including 'the rise and decline of the sole breadwinner role, declines in men's wages, and the flow of mothers into the paid labour force have altered normative roles for generations of men within families' (Roy, 2006: 31). As noted, the widespread entry of women into the labour market is perhaps the most striking aspect of these processes, shaping how both contemporary family and gender relations have been transformed in recent decades (Hanlon, 2012; Gray et al, 2016). Change in the economic organisation of gender roles is thought to have been accompanied by changing gendered attitudes that favour (and now necessitate) the sharing of income earning and homemaking (Gray et al, 2016). These new economic requirements have simultaneously impacted on the formation, stability and well-being of families and produced dramatic sociocultural reconstructions of masculinity and fatherhood (Henwood and Proctor, 2003). These changes are also reflected in the differing cultural expectations of younger generations of men today, which appear to be markedly different to those of their fathers (McDowell, 2003; Brannen and Nilsen, 2006; United Nations, 2011). The biographical research of Julia Brannen and colleagues (see Brannen and Nilsen, 2006; Brannen et al, 2011) is an important exemplar of these gradual generational shifts in normative expectations among men (see also Dermott and Miller, 2015; Brannen, 2019). The extent of generational change, Brannen and Nilsen (2006) suggest, is linked to the intersections of structural and cultural change and gender, although as considered in Chapter 2, the extent to which these are realised in practice may vary according to social class. As a major contribution to fatherhood research, Brannen and Nilsen's findings illustrate the value of exploring the factual side of fathers' biographies in historical context. Their sensitivity to men's biographical narratives in historical context transcends the structure–agency tension by combining knowledge of both individual and structural aspects of society; an approach taken up and applied in this book.

Recent global trend data reflects some positive evidence that change in men's practices is keeping pace with cultural change, although with national and regional variation. Global patterns reflect that there has been an overall increase in the time men spend on care activities (albeit still to a lesser extent than women, United Nations, 2011). This is linked to decreasing global fertility, which has increased men's time use and financial investment in children. The increasingly diverse patterns of repartnering and parenting described earlier in the chapter are also thought to be shaping the extent of men's involvements in fathering, producing increasingly complex patterns of family ties, responsibilities and care relations that are practised both within and across households and intergenerationally (Neale, 2000). Processes of marital breakdown through divorce, non-marital births and the separation of married or never-married couples with children have wrought further changes in the practice of relationships and parenthood, characterising the domestic landscape (Neale, 2000). An increased range of possibilities are being opened up by processes of family reformation linked to remarriage, the creation of reformed or step-families through repartnering, lone parenthood and parenting outside the boundaries of households, such as non-resident fatherhood (Bradshaw et al, 1999; Dermott, 2016; Neale and Patrick, 2016). These processes form the backdrop against which ideologies and ideals of 'good' and 'bad' fatherhood also evolve and that discursively constitute the modern paradox of father involvement and absence (discussed in Chapter 1). As noted, the 'new' ethos of engaged and involved fatherhood (Dermott, 2003; 2008), accompanied by increases in working motherhood and more progressive public ideals around gender equality, places greater emphasis on the significance of men's emotional and practical engagements in support for their children, as well as constructions of fathers as co-parents who share in parenting roles (Summers et al, 2006).

The extent to which the new ideology of engaged fatherhood is reflected in family practices as a material reality continues to be much debated in academic literatures, however (Dermott and Miller, 2015). Historically observed discrepancies between the images and practices of fatherhood call into question the extent of change and continuity in perceptions and ideologies related to fatherhood and what men (and women) do. While more women have entered the labour market there is limited evidence of an equivalent increase in men's involvement in unpaid labour and caregiving relative to women's workload (Daly and Rake, 2003). Segal (1990, 2006) captures this lag effectively in the title of her text *Slow Motion*, which describes the slow pace of change. Even despite the prevalence of models of involved and new fathers, parenting remains a gendered practice. The 'incomplete' or 'stalled' revolution (Hochschild, 1989) thesis maintains that transformations in gender relations in the domestic sphere continue to lag in comparison to other domains (see Miller, 2010a; Naldini et al, 2018). This thesis is supported by decades of research that confirms that the increasing participation of women in employment has not been accompanied by the reciprocal movement of men towards the embrace of domestic work and childcare. This has been delegated instead to low-paid, typically female workers or retained as an additional unpaid burden for women (Brooks and Hodkinson, 2020). The continued salience of the breadwinning model of fatherhood is also indicative that cultural ideologies have yet to be wholly influenced by changing gender patterns, deindustrialisation and patterns of unemployment (see Dolan, 2014; Morgan, 2003). The picture across national contexts is variable, however. Research about involved fatherhoods in the Nordic states suggests that involved fatherhood is more commonplace and thus both ideological and practised. In the UK, the picture is more fluid, such that it remains largely ideological and yet to be fully realised (Brannen and Nilsen, 2006).

While these patterns of difference across contexts indicate the coexistence and greater acceptance of different masculinities and models of fatherhood both in practice and in policies (Miller, 2010a), there is little evidence to suggest any wholesale transformation in gendered practices (Neale and Patrick, 2016, see also see van der Gaag et al, 2019). While fathers in the UK express a desire to 'be there' for their children, in practice, their contribution to childcare remains relatively small, as evidenced by the persistence of gender inequalities in the home that are experienced by women (Deutsch and Gaunt, 2020). Thus, while work–care arrangements have become more diverse and gendered ideologies and representations of parenthood have continually shifted over time, intergenerational continuities in traditional gendered divisions of labour are still apparent.

Recent literatures examining how gender ideologies held among couples change when they first transition to parenthood also reflect this position. There is evidence to suggest that relationships considered to be egalitarian in terms of gendered divisions of labour prior to having children often shift in the transition to parenthood, reflecting a more traditional gendered division of labour on the arrival of a child (for example, Miller, 2018a). Strongly ingrained and widely held assumptions that women are primarily responsible for childcare and domestic labour persist, constructing fathers as secondary or peripheral figures in caregiving. Today, adult manhood is still universally defined by societies, institutions, individuals and public policies through the role of provider, breadwinner and working man. These pervasive ideals also continue to be recognised among men as a core pillar of male identity and hegemonic masculinity, politically and culturally dominant constructions of masculinity (Dolan, 2014; Maxwell, 2018; Walker and Roberts, 2018). As Neale and Patrick (2016: 8) eloquently state, fathers are still more likely to 'start from an imperative to earn, while mothers start from an imperative to care'. An ongoing question therefore remains about the extent to which the symbolic aspects of gender identity in relation to involved fatherhood really constitute a move towards more egalitarian, nurturing masculinities or whether gendered styles of care/parenting continue to replicate aspects of traditional and/or hegemonic masculinity.

The gendered imperatives to earn or care are also reinforced to varying degrees by structural factors, including work–life balance policies and organisational cultures. The legislation of successive UK governments has ostensibly sought to encourage father involvement by strengthening fathers' responsibilities for their children, regardless of marital or residential status, through provisions like shared parenting or paternal leave (Neale and Patrick, 2016, see also Haywood and Johansson, 2017). Paradoxically, though, these changes remain premised on constructions of men as employees, financial providers and breadwinners. While there have been encouraging shifts to support men and women in the reconciliation of economic provisioning and the daily care of families (Burgess and Davies, 2017; also see Maxwell, 2018), policy still tends to emphasise men's roles in providing 'cash rather than care'[2] (Featherstone, 2009; United Nations, 2011; Yarwood, 2011; Meah and Jackson, 2016). In the American context, which has pursued comparable policy approaches to the UK, stereotypes about dead-beat dads who fail to earn are similarly codified in welfare reform legislation through a strengthened focus on child support enforcement rather than time spent with children (Summers et al, 2006; see also Eisenstadt and Oppenheim, 2019; Featherstone, 2009 for UK reforms to child maintenance). The promotion of models of 'work-focussed' fathering in policy mean that it is perhaps unsurprising that men continue to uphold male breadwinning as a central tenet of good fatherhood (Shirani et al, 2012).

Theorising masculinities and fatherhoods in transition

Debates about the tensions men navigate between expectations of breadwinning and caregiving, either as fathers or as family caregivers, are often tied to wider discussions about modern masculinities, which are theorised as being 'in transition' (Williams, 2009; Roberts, 2018). The work of Raewyn Connell (1995), which she later updated with Messerschmidt (2005), has been especially significant for theorising masculinities as socially constructed and relational and for demonstrating the multiplicity of masculinities and their differing configurations. Her framework of multiple masculinities illustrates the plurality of masculinities while also sustaining focus on the gender order, which maintains privilege for men over women but may also enable and/or constrain some men in different ways (Williams, 2009). In the now classic text, *Masculinities*, Connell (1995) refined the concept of hegemonic masculinity, defining it as a variety of masculinity that is relationally configured and hierarchical, positioned with and against complicit, marginalised (for example, poor working-class men and ethnic minorities) and subordinated (for example, sexual minorities) masculinities, and in relation to women (see also Tarrant and Ward, 2020). Connell's framework of multiple masculinities therefore offers a complex theory of masculinities that maintains a focus on power relations and acknowledges them as collective (as well as individual), actively constructed, internally complex and subject to change over time and space (Connell, 2010). Also captured are men's individual capacities for change and development, as well as the intersectional nature of identities, including their inextricable links with other forms of social inequalities such as class, age and generation (Hopkins and Noble, 2009; King and Calasanti, 2013). As major factors in the social construction of masculinity, social categories like ethnicity, class, sexuality and age interact with gender in often complex and contradictory ways to produce varied and unequally valued positionalities (Slutskaya et al, 2016).

Connell's work therefore articulates a more dynamic view of masculinities, arguing that they are always open to challenge, contest and change. Social geographical scholarship has advanced the argument that, rather than a fixed, unitary and natural concept, masculinities have an inherently spatial character and are 'constituted by an amalgam of practices, values and meanings and realised in particular places and contexts' (Hopkins and Noble, 2009: 813). This diversity is also encompassed in temporal and processual understandings of masculinities and fatherhoods that conceptualise them as in transition (for example, Robinson and Hockey, 2011; Johansson and Andreasson, 2018; Roberts, 2018). Informed by concepts of time and temporality, we are better able to conceive of masculinities as fluid and changeable; to understand men and social change; and to recognise men as capable of change over the lifecourse. In fatherhood research, this increased theoretical sophistication has generated a shift from one-off 'snapshots' of men characteristic of much research on fatherhood and masculinities (Neale and Flowerdew, 2003) to a 'moving picture' of fatherhood (Miller, 2018b).

The notion of a moving picture resonates with arguments developed by Robinson and Hockey (2011), who capture this fluidity in men's individual lifecourses by conceptualising their participants as 'men in motion'. Their research is attentive to the open-ended and processual nature of masculinities (and fatherhood) and how men perform these aspects of their identities differently, across the various spheres of their life and at different times across the lifecourse. Conceptually, transitions capture both change and continuities, so that the boundaries between public and private arenas can be seen to be constituted differently for men and women of different ages and social class backgrounds (Whitehead, 2002; Robinson and Hockey, 2011).

The extent and veracity of these transitions remain in question, with recognition that men variously negotiate more traditional ideologies of masculinity alongside what have been termed softer, more 'inclusive masculinities' (a well-recognised but contested concept) (for example, Anderson, 2009) and caring masculinities that are thought to demonstrate a shift in attitudes and practices (Ward, 2015b). More recently, there have been concerted efforts to integrate masculinities studies with feminist ethics-of-care perspectives to theorise this ostensible progression towards *caring masculinities* (Hanlon, 2012; Elliott, 2016). Elliott's (2016: 241) practice-based model suggests that the central features of caring masculinities 'are their rejection of domination and their integration of values of care, such as positive emotion, interdependence and relationality, into masculine identities'. Stemming mainly from studies of fatherhood, the analysis of caring masculinities is considered to have the dual value of demonstrating empirically that men are capable of care, and theoretically, how hegemonic notions of masculinities can be destabilised via care (Jordan, 2020b). Unpaid and family care are important arenas in which the doing of alternative masculinities can transgress stereotypical constructions of men and care work (Milligan and Morbey, 2016). According to Milligan and Morbey (2016: 108), care work is thought to 'loosen men's identity formations within the limits of hegemonic masculinity, opening up opportunities for alternative ways of "being male" and resisting hegemonic masculinity norms'.

The shift towards theorising changing or evolving masculinities (for example, Richards Solomon, 2017) as inherently caring is not unproblematic, however. In defining practices of fathering as 'new' or in transition, there is a risk of perhaps inadvertently erasing the histories of men's family participation. I suggest that this is a limitation of current gender analyses. Despite being temporally oriented to capture an ostensible shift towards men becoming more caring, the idea that care was ever beyond the boundaries of masculinities is problematic in and of itself and is not empirically supported in either historical or contemporary research with men as fathers. Notwithstanding the raft of research about contemporary fatherhoods, the social-historical evidence presented in Chapter 2 illustrates effectively that men have always engaged in caring practices and family participation, and, indeed, so have women in household economies as a form of employment (Doucet, 2020). 'Men-as-father has always been subsumed under the history of pervasive patriarchy', as Laqueur (1990: 205, cited by Doucet, 2020: 2) notes, and by the deficit perspectives of fathering identified in Chapter 1 that judge men as inadequate parents.

Attempts to generalise about fathers across time are therefore problematic, especially given the sparsity of evidence (Brannen and Nilsen, 2006). Despite a burgeoning of contributions to the evidence base, including by social historians, continued limitations in conceptual language also add to this challenge. Doucet (2020) takes this analysis further, suggesting that beyond the emphasis on what fathers do as caring, we need narratives of fatherhood that attend to the complex entanglements of breadwinning and caregiving and that adequately capture the conceptual and practice-based interplay between the two. There is a risk with the concept of caring masculinities that it becomes ahistoric, especially in its premise that masculinities are in some way evolving towards care. There are also viable concerns that caring masculinity may be co-opted and become a 'new hegemon' in ways that bolster the patriarchal order (Jordan, 2020b). Jordan (2020b), for example, introduces some necessary caution about how the concept may be mobilised. Drawing on a case study of the UK-based Fathers4Justice activist group, she foregrounds the need to pay careful attention to the contexts in which caring masculinities may be employed, in both strategic and problematic ways that reflect anti-feminist values.

These critiques indicate a heightened need for recognition that men are, and always have been, capable of care, as well as further evidence about how such engagements in care might be both recognised and supported to flourish in ways that promote progress towards gender equality (for example, Boyer et al, 2017; Tarrant, 2018). Cultural models of involved fatherhood are empirically grounded on the archetypal experiences and practices of white, middle-class men, yet the conditions and expectations for involved fatherhood are additionally shaped by social class, as well as economic, social and cultural capital (Edwards et al, 2015; Bedston et al, 2019). Moreover, these debates confirm the need for an intersectional analysis within groups of men so as to understand how disadvantages and inequalities affect whom family participation is most accessible to, and why. Age, for example, is a cross-cutting issue, with young, disadvantaged men identified as being most at risk of becoming disconnected from work and family life, the key markers of successful male adulthood (Roy et al, 2015). While economic recessionary processes, labour market change and unemployment may produce opportunities for men to reconfigure their parental and personal identities (Smith, 2009) in ways that reinforce sociocultural expectations around female breadwinning households and men sharing in care work (Boyer et al, 2017; see also Chapter 2), there is still a need to understand how a progressive regendering of care processes can be promoted and sustained at a structural level so that those who choose to engage in family care are not penalised.

Notable here is that the effects of these radical societal shifts in economic and gender relations are not felt evenly; they impact negatively on some family arrangements, more so than on others, with potential to preclude transformative opportunities for fathers located at the margins. Based on qualitative research with fathers in precarious employment circumstances in Slovenia, for example, Hrženjak (2017) is critical of the way in which involved fatherhood is often constructed as an issue of men's individual identity change and rising awareness among families that gender equality and family well-being can be achieved through more egalitarian models of parenting and homemaking. She argues that these assumptions obscure the contextual factors (that is, the broader structures, policies and organisations) that enable or constrain the progress and possibilities of individual change in fatherhood practices (Hrženjak, 2017). Evidence suggests that work–life balance appears to be much more achievable for men in countries where welfare and organisational support is generally less conditional, for example. Further empirical evidence is therefore required about how men's experiences are variously shaped, and marginalised, by different dimensions of social identity and inequality and what kinds of broader policy, welfare and organisational interventions facilitate men's caregiving or prevent it from flourishing. Such an approach decentres questions of whether and how men as individuals are or are not caring (an approach based on an individualisation thesis) and instead emphasises the need to understand the broader relational and processual dynamics that contour the lives of men located in the margins.

Masculinities and the doing of kinship

The previous sections have demonstrated that both families and men and masculinities are in a transformational period and that the plural character of masculinities is also present in families. As Genest Dufault and Castelain Meunier (2017) note, the relationship between 'men and the family is particularly complex as it is located at an intersection of several aspects including: identity, relations, institutions and politics'. The ostensible emancipation of women from intimate and domestic spheres through their integration into the workforce, accompanied by new models of father involvement, has generated renewed interest in the reproduction of unequal power relations between men and women in the everyday, micro-level practices of 'doing family' (Morgan, 1996). Of note here, theoretically, is that family relationships can be seen to contribute to the doing (and undoing) of gender, including how gender is produced and reproduced in everyday life and, along with other social (in)equalities, comes to be transmitted to new generations (West and Zimmerman, 1987; Naldini et al, 2018). From this perspective both family and gender are conceptualised as accomplishments, achieved through practices, structures and norms both inside and outside the domestic sphere. Making an explicit link, Comas d'Argemir and Soronellas (2019) argue that changes in gender and kinship relations are interconnected processes.

A broad feminist literature that has examined care as labour provides fertile ground for considering these interrelations. Highlighting the complexity of care as a concept, Comas d'Argemir and Soronellas (2019) identify an interdisciplinary scholarship that emphasises both the affective and moral (Gilligan, 1982; Finch and Groves, 1983; Tronto, 1993) and social and material dimensions (Daly and Lewis, 2000; Glenn, 2010) inherent in relationships of care. Care is distinctly gendered and is often accorded low social value. It can also involve the doing of kinship, however, as Comas d'Argemir and Soronellas (2019) argue. While research on care has highlighted the role of gender, it has largely been blind to the links between care and kinship. They suggest that when women provide care they often do so because they are mothers, wives, daughters and relatives by marriage. As Finch and Mason (1993) argue (see also Doucet, 2018), caring for others is intricately connected to people's identities as moral beings, and what it means to be a good father, a generous mother, a caring sister and so on is worked out from within a social and cultural location and with reference to others. Generational and familial identities are therefore a constituent element of care (Comas d'Argemir and Soronellas, 2019). Furthering their analysis, Comas d'Argemir and Soronellas (2019: 316) argue that,

> like gender, kinship is a social and cultural product that distributes roles and responsibilities and places them within a hierarchy. Not everyone with the same kinship relationship is equally involved in care, meaning that as in gender dynamics, it is necessary to understand how kinship roles are negotiated and transformed, changing the sense of duty and reciprocity attributed to them.

Based on their research with men in Catalonia, Spain, Comas d'Argemir and Soronellas (2019) explain that men are increasingly becoming new agents in care linked to a twofold crisis of care and economy. They first elaborate the care crisis, which refers to the collapse of family and society's ability to meet increasing demands for care, compounded by the fragmentation of family networks and change in gendered and intergenerational relations discussed earlier in this chapter. Second, they explain that the global economic crisis and austerity have deeply and disproportionately impacted on families that lack the socioeconomic resources required to access market-led services. This, they suggest, has increased the need for men's involvement in family care. Focusing on men's family participation through their accounts as active participants in family life and framing them as about doing kinship is therefore significant for advancing understanding of the complex links between masculinities, kinship and caring; the extent to which intergenerational and gendered change engender the renegotiation and redistribution of care roles and responsibilities within family contexts; and how, why and when men participate in family care.

They also argue that barriers to men's involvement in care are both cultural and related to opportunity. With distinct parallels with arguments established in fatherhood research, men who provide family care are confronted with cultural barriers 'based on the assimilation of care as something that women do and on hegemonic masculinity' (Connell, 1995; Connell and Messerschmidt, 2005 cited by Comas d'Argemir and Soronellas, 2019: 318). Barriers to opportunity are linked to the wage and job differences afforded to men and women (Comas d'Argemir and Soronellas, 2019). Nevertheless, in invoking the doing of kinship, men who provide care, for example, as elderly men to their wives or partners, or as grandfathers, continually navigate the tensions of caregiving through complicity, if not adherence, to hegemonic masculinity (Mann et al, 2016).

Theorising low-income family life and local ties

So far, the discussions in this chapter have considered the dynamic and relational character of masculinities and familial practices. In the final section of the chapter, contemporary theorising about low-income family life and local ties are considered. In Chapter 2 it is noted that the experiences of men who father or engage in father-like relationships in contexts of poverty and disadvantage have received limited empirical attention from social scientists, although there is evidence to suggest that unemployment and marginalisation can lead to gender-role strain and the breakdown of social relations for men. An overemphasis on pessimistic outcomes makes it harder to conceive of the possibility that marginalised masculinities can be transformative and that marginalised men might also have the capacity to perform caring masculinities.

Daly and Kelly (2015) go as far as to suggest that family life under conditions of poverty has been theorised inadequately, especially when compared with the development of theories of poverty and their application within household studies. Nevertheless, there are notable British and international studies of low-income motherhood (for example, Gillies, 2007; Jensen, 2018), low-income grandparenthood (Hughes and Emmel, 2011) and families living in low-income circumstances (for example, Desmond, 2012; Daly and Kelly, 2015) which indicate the value of sociological explorations of the longitudinal dynamics of family life in low-income contexts. The key features of some of these contributions are elaborated in what follows with consideration of their relevance for advancing understanding of men's interdependencies in low-income families and contexts.

Sociological research has long been concerned with questions of how low-income and destitute families endure crises, including how they supplement their incomes by relying on kinship networks. American sociologist Desmond (2012) traces these interests back to the pioneering studies of Engels in Manchester (1845) and Booth in London (1902–4) in the UK, and outlines a notable body of research in the American context that evidences the saliency of extensive kin and friendship networks as key to the survival of urban poor communities marked by severe economic deprivation (for example, Du Bois, 1899; Stack, 1974, cited by Desmond, 2012). More recent debates question the centrality of kin support and the extent to which the poor rely on mutual support among family members and friends to survive (Desmond, 2012). These literatures demonstrate how low-income families are often embedded in small and dense networks within the communities in which they live and work but also suggest that ties are often infused with mistrust and non-cooperation rather than kin solidarity and mutual cooperation (Desmond, 2012).

To address this divergence of views, Desmond (2012) sought to evaluate the degree to which families experiencing eviction from their homes in high-poverty neighbourhoods in the US depended on their family and friends. He identified a mix of family practices and activities ranging from extended family support to hospital visits, family reunions and funerals. These sit alongside the withholding of family support altogether. In his study and in the absence of family ties, families relied instead on disposable ties with acquaintances. These relatively fleeting ties were characterised by high physical co-presence, reciprocal or semi-reciprocal exchanges of resources and an accelerated intimacy. Interestingly, male family members and descriptions of their family participation feature heavily in the empirical accounts presented by Desmond but their contributions are not foregrounded, perhaps because his arguments are less attentive to questions of gender.

In British sociology and social policy it is well established that lone mothers who are well embedded in a fabric of social support are likely to be less vulnerable to adverse circumstances and are more likely to rely on personal relationships of care as a buffer (Klett-Davies, 2007; Millar and Ridge, 2009; Canton, 2018). Similarly, the Teesside studies, which sought to explore popular poverty myths around intergenerational cultures of worklessness and cultures of poverty located in specific families and localities (MacDonald et al, 2005), discovered the significance of being embedded in local family and extended support networks for mediating some of the more negative local effects of problems like drug use and criminal victimisation.

Another important contribution to the theorisation of the relationship between families and poverty is the family vulnerability literature. Where the masculinities literature has examined the social contexts that marginalise some men (see previous sections), marginalisation in family studies has been conceptualised in terms of vulnerabilities. While the cultural theorisation of the relationship between family and poverty emphasises moral dispositions and discourses as causal explanations for poverty, structural explanations indicate family structures that are more 'at risk' of vulnerability, particularly as expressed through policy contexts (Daly, 2018). Indeed, the normative nuclear family as a self-sufficient and independent unit is often considered to be the most effective for raising children (Chambers, 2012). Capitalist societies incentivise traditional families while impoverishing and undermining 'actual' or non-traditional families. The concept of family vulnerability captures the multiple aspects that render families vulnerable, involving the following, overlapping dimensions (Mynarska et al, 2015: 9):

1. economic difficulties/lack of financial resources: poverty, low living standards, housing problems (for example, too damp, too expensive, too cold or difficult to heat);
2. social exclusion: limited access to facilities such as shops, schools, libraries or medical services;
3. lack of (or limited), social support from social networks: no assistance from family members, friends, neighbours or colleagues (referring to practical help as well as emotional support);
4. stigmatisation: being a victim of stereotypes, being devalued, confronted with disgraceful behaviour because of belonging to a particular social or ethnic group;

5. health difficulties: disadvantages resulting from poor mental health, physical health or disabilities;
6. being a victim of crime: in the family context, especially of violence.

A combination of these dimensions was apparent in the narratives of the participants in the MPLC study. Social policy and wider macro-level developments have an important role to play in reducing the reproduction of family vulnerability (namely poverty) over time and across generations. According to Mynarska et al (2015), family well-being should be predicated on a comprehensive policy strategy and suite of measures that support families in a sustainable manner achieved via a combination of education and employment support and the creation of a family-friendly society. This might include reconciliation policies that support the ability of men and women to combine earning and caring; enable adequate access to education from the early years onwards; and sustainable funding and availability of social support services, particularly for the most disadvantaged families. Recognising care as an integral aspect of the social infrastructure is essential to this vision and stands in distinction to individualising policies that are premised on gendered ideological models and assumptions about fatherlessness (see Chapter 1).

Dynamic research has been described as providing the most comprehensive understanding of poverty because it is able to record stories of change over time as opposed to point-in-time studies, which provide a 'snap-shot' view (Smith and Middleton, 2009). The dynamic view of poverty counters the idea of a single, homogeneous experience by demonstrating the mechanisms that influence how and why individuals move back and forth across the poverty line over time and how different social groups experience it. As argued in Chapter 2, gender inequalities affect poverty risks and act as a mediating influence on routes in and out of poverty (Bennett and Daly, 2014). Additionally, both the type of household and family that an individual lives in can affect poverty risks, while the distribution of caring and family responsibilities both within and across households affects access to resources over the lifecourse (Bennett and Daly, 2014).

Perhaps the most comprehensive contribution to theoretical developments in understanding the dynamic relationship between family and poverty is that elaborated by Daly and Kelly (2015), mentioned earlier. Their framework captures both the structural and agentic dimensions of family poverty and advances an experiential understanding, that is, how families respond to the situation of having a low income and the actions they take (Daly and Kelly, 2015).

They propose a focus on family life for understanding the dynamics of poverty, for two reasons. One is that families are an important arrangement of personal life; the second is that people tend to live and define themselves in families rather than households. Daly and Kelly (2015) identify that resource distributions and familial well-being are more than just economic fact; they are mediated and filtered through the complex relationships, norms and practices that people associate with family. They propose and apply a theoretical framework that suggests attentiveness to four main elements, including:

- family as structure and mode of organisation (a structural approach that recognises how the composition and organisation of family affects access to and decisions around resources);
- cultural specificity, meaning and identity (how people interpret their situation in the context of social norms and values);
- relationships, activities and processes (here the concept of 'family practices' (Morgan, 2011) is a useful lens, as it captures the sets of activities associated with maintaining and governing family life);
- family as object of public representation and local life (namely that the self and family need to be constantly created and recreated, especially in public life).

A key aim of this book is to examine and understand family poverty and its associated hardships via a social and relational lens (Ridge, 2009) that is attentive to men's caring arrangements and how their family participation is shaped by the conditions of living on a low income. Relational lenses like these capture the complex textures of poverty as they permeate family lives, as well as the variable facets and impacts of deprivation as they play out in everyday contexts, circumstances and family relationships. In this framework, participants are also positioned as subjects rather than objects of research and their voices are foregrounded rather than subsumed.

Concluding remarks

As noted in the introductory chapter, a key aim of this book is to move beyond the prurient and binary focus on father absence, presence and preoccupation with crisis in paternal roles, and towards a more dynamic conceptualisation of men's family participation, constituting a key theoretical contribution to the field. Doing so involves seeing men as active participants in their family lives and intergenerational relations, including in contexts of low income. Despite men's experiences of low-income life being an area of empirical neglect, this chapter has situated MPLC in these broader bodies of theoretical and substantive knowledge. They not only informed the original focus of enquiry for the study, but also have application to its findings.

This framework elaborates the complex, dynamic and intersectional relationships between masculinities, family and low-income life and encompasses several thematic considerations including the everyday doing of masculinities, kinship and care; intergenerational exchanges (material, emotional and care based) both within families and across households; the patterning of gendered and generational interdependencies and caregiving over time; and the influence of economic and material deprivation on these processes. These bodies of work not only apply to the MPLC findings but are also advanced, and indeed in some cases confirmed and refined, by the new insights produced by the study, to which the next chapter now turns.

4

Supporting men in low-income contexts: practitioner observations

A significant context in which men in low-income families negotiate their identities as 'present' fathers is in encounters with health and social care services. It is in these contexts that family tensions and disputes in relation to men's roles, responsibilities and rights in connection with their children coalesce, are supported, refuted and sometimes denied (Tarrant and Hughes, 2019). In the first of the empirical chapters of the book, accounts are presented of men's family participation and complex needs as observed by local welfare providers and professionals in the city where the MPLC study was conducted. These accounts render visible the local and national practice and policy contexts contouring men's participation in low-income families and localities and develop an understanding of the (inter)dependencies of men with local services and providers. The findings confirm that marginalised men are most visible to services when they are seeking to secure resources on behalf of their families or in relation to the individual troubles they may experience, such as material deprivation, problems securing employment and/or physical and mental health problems.

The analyses presented in this chapter are interpretations of data generated from informal ethnographic conversations, semi-structured interviews and a knowledge-exchange workshop held with several professionals to share early findings from the secondary analysis work that was conducted using existing data about low-income men (see Chapter 1 and Appendix 2). The professionals who agreed to participate were at the coal-face of changing family patterns and had an accumulated wealth of knowledge about the problems men encounter in their personal and family lives. The findings illustrate the importance of local networks of formal support for families living in hardship, as well as how professionals interpret and respond to men's experiences of marginalisation and disadvantage. Notably, it was service providers working for third sector and voluntary agencies who demonstrated a keen awareness and understanding of the complex needs and experiences of marginalised men and their families in the city. They also interpreted the experiences of the men with whom they were engaging within the policy frameworks and discourses that framed them. The contextual features they describe offer an additional layer of understanding about the local processes and contexts that variously impact on men's family participation and that work to sustain or mitigate against it. To provide context to the findings, the chapter begins with a brief overview of a burgeoning body of research evidence that examines the gendered character of family and parenting support and the dependencies of low-income families on local and regulatory agencies and services.

Low-income family interdependencies on services

MPLC sought to research men who are simultaneously 'visible' through media and political scrutiny and to regulatory agencies, yet 'invisible' in terms of their limited ability to actively consent to engagements with regulatory processes voluntarily because they have complex needs (Emmel et al, 2007; Hemmerman, 2010). Longitudinal research with low-income families (Emmel and Hughes, 2010) and young fathers (Neale and Davies, 2015b) has demonstrated the vital role that services provide in enabling fathers' access to resources on behalf of their families and to address vulnerabilities. However, failures by professionals to work effectively with fathers have also proven to be resistant and long standing (Philip et al, 2018) and may also contribute to the absenting of men from families via practices of surveillance and sidelining (Neale et al, 2015).

Our previous analyses of men in low-income families and contexts indicate the importance both of legal systems and support services in either ameliorating or exacerbating vulnerability in the lives of low-income men and families (Tarrant and Hughes, 2019). Like all families, low-income families benefit from economic stability, safety, good health and community engagement. However, the complexities of their lives are greatly impacted by limited economic resource. Support services, including those that are locally embedded in communities, provide access to crucial resources for people's everyday needs, including those that enable low-income families to flourish (Emmel et al, 2007; Neale et al, 2015). Yet seeking and getting help, as well as processes of accessing health and social care services, is rarely straightforward for people whose lives reflect a range of complex needs and uncertainties (Hughes and Emmel, 2011).

These contextual constraints may be further compounded for men who are fathers by the gendered landscape of support. Where support and/or services are not available or where professionals engage in a 'risk'-based approach to men as fathers (Neale and Davies, 2015b), families are often exposed to 'shocks' that have the potential to tip them even further into crisis (Emmel and Hughes, 2014). While men are lesser known for turning to professionals for assistance, depending on their level of need and/or resource, men with care responsibilities can still be expected to encounter a broad range of public services along their parenting and even grandparenting journeys. This includes ante-natal and maternity services, education and early years settings, employment services and/or housing and custody support (Tarrant and Neale, 2017a). The child protection system, criminal justice system and services designed to support men with domestic abuse are also areas where low-income families and fathers are encountered and worked with (Maxwell et al, 2012; Bulman and Neale, 2017; Morris et al, 2018). Third and voluntary sector organisations with a specific remit to support families and individuals with complex needs also often provide essential resources when they are available.

As Philip et al (2018) note in their discussion of men's recurrent experiences of the child protection system, the difficult economic circumstances of family life in the UK have implications for men as carers. They suggest that the child protection context has proven inadequate for accounting for economic hardship and places a disproportionate burden on those that are already marginalised or experiencing deprivation (Philip et al, 2018). This is confirmed by Bywaters et al (2016), who illustrate international evidence that deprivation is the largest contributory factor in children's chances of being looked after. Notwithstanding the multifaceted and evolving context through which working inclusively with fathers and male carers has become a necessity, these discussions emphasise the importance of professional encounters with fathers and wider adult male carers. Philips et al (2018) argue that there is a clear remit for working in collaboration with families via a relationship- and strengths-based approach and one that avoids binary assessments of fathers as either risk or resource.

These arguments reflect that encounters with health and social care services are not necessarily uncomplicated or always unproblematic for men (Tarrant and Hughes, 2019). A key issue is that mainstream preventative services often fail to engage fathers and many men perceive services as feminised and therefore irrelevant to them (Katz et al, 2007). Citing Bowlby et al (2010), Conlon et al (2014: 732) note that 'points at which formal and informal care "bump up" against each other are spaces managed and occupied primarily by women'. Research about specialist support groups for fathers also suggests that men often experience parenting provisions as gendered and report feeling marginalised by the perceived power of women who are more likely to occupy these spaces (Hanna, 2018). Social interventions for fathers are also a contested territory and may be affected by fraught gender politics underscored by debates between feminist and men's rights perspectives (Scourfield et al, 2014).

Negative or stereotypical attitudes towards fathers that may be held by professionals also represent a significant barrier to appropriate support and impact on how public services engage with men at the local level. In child protection contexts, professionals continue to be troubled by engagements with men, reflected in fearful and inflexible thinking by social workers about their roles in families and their presence in family homes (Philip et al, 2018). Gendered thinking by professionals, differing ideological perspectives on men's involvements, the female-centric nature of many services that work to support parents and families, allied with wider cultural assumptions that mothers remain primary caregivers (Neale and Patrick, 2016; Philip et al, 2018) are consequently pervasive issues. These complexities mean that men often remain on the periphery of service delivery (Tarrant and Neale, 2017a).

A more concerted effort by child and family services to work with fathers is a relatively recent development but is under-researched (Scourfield et al, 2014). There is compelling evidence to suggest, though, that shifts towards father involvement might be more achievable when driven at the level of practice and support (Tarrant and Neale, 2017a, 2017b). A recent synthesis of research literature summarising what works best in practice to support fathers and male adult carers is a useful resource for considering what services might do to engage men more effectively and in ways that promote father-inclusive approaches driven by a commitment to achieving gender equality (Tarrant and Neale, 2017a). Pockets of good practice in evidence across the UK suggest that the implementation of relatively small and cost-effective changes within services may engender a system change that recognises, values and encourages positive forms of involvement by men in children's lives (Tarrant and Neale, 2017a). Caring and compassionate approaches from workers and feeling cared for are especially important here (Featherstone et al, 2017; Tarrant and Neale, 2017a). Effective engagement relies on the development of quality relationships with men who access services; relationships that are established by workers who contest deficit thinking, recognise men's capabilities to care and make time to understand the troubles men face as situated in a broader context of social change. The professionals who participated in the MPLC research were especially attuned to the troubles expressed by the marginalised men whom they were supporting (some of whom agreed to become MPLC study participants) and offered important accounts of the local policy and practice context.

Researching with service providers and support professionals

The decision to map and consult with local third and voluntary sector professionals, as well as local authority personnel with responsibilities for delivering local policy priorities, was informed by several factors. Driven by an ethos of co-production and collaborative research practice, which was a central tenet of the research design for MPLC, the study sought to establish productive partnerships with non-academic professionals and actors. This kind of methodology has become increasingly important in recent years and somewhat of a normative expectation for social sciences research (Hall and Hiteva, 2020). The partnership working was driven by the intention to develop a responsive research approach to gaps in evidence around the value of developing and establishing inclusive support for men and fathers, both in the city where MPLC took place and nationally. Existing research suggests that men from low-income contexts are likely to have an extensive set of support needs, producing dependencies on a range of statutory and specialist support services. These men are therefore likely to engage with a wide variety of agencies at different times in their parenting journeys and in relation to different dimensions of their lives (Emmel and Hughes, 2010; Neale and Davies, 2015b). Engagements with professionals in MPLC were productive encounters from which we all learnt from one another to advance knowledge and understanding of an under-researched and poorly evidenced research area. As well as enabling access to participants, privileged insights were afforded about the specific practice and policy contexts shaping and affecting the lives of marginalised men in the city. Their accounts also confirmed that there were men in low-income families providing significant amounts of care, some of whom were themselves seeking support to address personal hardships.

The collaborative process comprised three methods: informal conversations that helped to establish trust and rapport, one-off individual semi-structured interviews and a knowledge-exchange workshop that brought a group of professionals together and provided an opportunity to share knowledge and prompt reflections on existing data pertaining to men's support needs. The semi-structured interviews, which were conducted with seven professionals from local services and the council, were designed to develop an understanding of the local policy context and support provision for men in the city; to ensure that the research would produce data with practical application for policy and practice; and to identify and negotiate access to participants. The questions that structured the individual interviews were wide ranging but predominantly centred on the role of the individual in their organisation; how they and the organisation might benefit from the MPLC research; organisational structure; current goals and ambitions of the organisation; collaborations with other organisations; how low-income men might benefit from the service; how far the service met the needs of low-income men; and how MPLC might produce impact for the men and families who participated.

The knowledge-exchange workshop had linked but distinctive goals. As a bridge between the findings emerging from the FYF and IGE datasets (mentioned in Chapter 1 and see Appendix 2) and the new phase of research with low-income fathers, the workshop was a collegiate space through which the professionals were able to forge new connections, share their experiences of good practice and debate key gaps in provision and policy agendas. Five members of local organisations attended the workshop and four of the attendees were those who had also been interviewed individually. The attendees were voluntary and third sector workers whose offer involved support for men experiencing deprivation and had orientations to men's identities as fathers or father figures. They therefore represented individuals and organisations working with men of all ages across the city. The specific roles and interests of these participants is described later in the chapter.

The outcomes of this workshop influenced the developing design of the MPLC study, which was well placed to respond flexibly to evidence gaps identified by local services and enable the generation of relevant findings. Working closely with professionals from a range of support agencies in the city confirmed not only the prevalence of men in low-income families engaging in otherwise invisible caregiving but also that local civil society was a vital lifeline for some men in enabling them to support and resource their families and adapt to personal crisis and periods of familial and intergenerational change. The discussions therefore revealed some of the barriers that men were facing and seeking support for, as well as how services themselves were responding to men's needs. Insights from the professionals who were interviewed and who participated at the workshop are analysed in the remainder of the chapter following a brief overview of the demographic characteristics of the city where MPLC took place.

A brief note on the city as context

It is worth noting here that the new qualitative insights generated about the local policy context via this process overlaid existing and emerging quantitative evidence about the rapidly changing socioeconomic context of the city at the time of the study. By 2008, the city had become the second-largest finance and business centre in the UK outside of London. However, the global financial crisis caused a sharp decline in both manufacturing and finance jobs. The Joint Strategic Needs Assessment for the city in 2015 indicated that worklessness, financial exclusion, impacts of poor housing on health, poor educational attainment and reduced life chances were concentrated in specific localities of the city. The most deprived communities in the Inner East and Inner South areas of the city were where many of the study participants were known to these professionals and were recruited from. A recent report on the state of men's health in the city (not cited for ethical reasons) indicates that, of the 368,000 males residing in the city, 2,000 are single parents with dependent children; around 6,000 are of working age and provide 20 hours or more of unpaid care; they are more likely than women to die younger; and they are more likely to lead unhealthy lives, especially in less affluent areas. While such figures provide important evidence of the broader statistical picture they offer only a partial account. The professionals interviewed were able to reflect on their own engagements with men with care responsibilities in low-income localities and were keen to understand more about the qualitative experiences of men and their engagements with services to affect change in practice and inform policy.

Formal agencies

Three individuals from the local authority were interviewed; one was a manager of a team that supported kinship carers and two, who were interviewed together, were involved in implementing a city-wide policy initiative prompted by the national 'Troubled Families' agenda. In this city, there was an evident commitment to fostering a relational approach to thinking about and working with families. The narratives of these formal agencies reflected the pro-family legislative backdrop of the UK and a child welfare context that seeks permanency for children when they are no longer able to reside with birth parents (Cooper, 2013) by keeping them in family contexts. Government policy, since the Children Act 1989 stipulates that the first option for the care of a child should be a member of the extended family or social network, in the event of parental incapacity (Hunt and Waterhouse, 2012).

Proposing to offer a more coordinated and supportive approach to families, the two local authority workers who were interviewed together were keen to examine early intervention approaches in support for children that recognised the unique circumstances of their family contexts, acknowledged the strengths and resources of those families and that were attentive to where additional support might be necessary. Highlighting attempts to establish a coordinated policy approach they explained: "Our issue really in trying to promote this [policy initiative] stuff is to challenge the other boards to say, actually, if you want decent outcomes for kids, you've got to support adults with vulnerability. That's where we're really trying to get evidence." Interestingly, their arguments around supporting adults with vulnerability, while well founded and attentive to wider family dynamics, were also underscored by reference to cycles of deprivation and worklessness. The existence of intergenerational cycles of worklessness has largely been debunked in contemporary sociological research. A recent mixed-methods study by Shildrick et al (2012), for example, that was developed to identify families who were workless across three or more generations using statistical data, was unable to find any multi-generational workless families. It identified much more complex patterns of recurrent poverty within families instead. The longitudinal ethnography conducted by Coffield et al (1980) between 1975 and 1978 also critiqued these ideas over four decades ago, yielding detailed biographies of families experiencing multiple deprivations. This study highlighted a much more complex web of factors that could lead families in or out of poverty. While the socioeconomic conditions of the UK have rapidly shifted since then (see Chapter 3), the tendency to blame families and characterise them as workless in policy is a notable continuity. Despite being subject to sustained academic critique, these ideas were nonetheless driving local council priorities for ensuring better outcomes for children, demonstrating how cultural thinking informs the views of professionals:

> 'We know from our cohorts with the troubled families that it's all intergenerational, worklessness. So, the young lads that are on it, their parents won't have worked and their parents probably won't have worked, and there'll be multiple issues.
>
> 'One of the big ones is the [name of initiative to support the wider family], so the idea of that is for practitioners, whoever they're working with, whether you're a family worker, a probation worker just working with adults, youth

offending, just working with young people, a nursery nurse, whoever it is, you need to be looking at the needs of the wider family and how their needs are impacting upon your client.'

These comments highlight an important and much-needed commitment towards the need for professionals to identify and work with wider family members beyond households to understand and support those who first engage with services. However, other research indicates that it is often rare for services to work beyond the family, meaning that critical family members, including fathers, can fall through the net if family circumstances or needs change (Morris et al, 2017). Furthermore, Neale and Davies (2015b) note in their focus on the support needs of young fathers that when organisations and services lead with negative and stigmatising perceptions of individuals and their families, such as those indicated here in relation to the presumption of intergenerational worklessness, this can cause suspicion, affect trust and become a major barrier to engagement and partnership working.

The council's kinship care support team were able to provide more detailed accounts of men in low-income family contexts and proved to be a relatively successful route for accessing older adult males for the study. At the time of the interview the team were doing a lot of work to improve their offer of support for carers in the city and were interested in understanding more about the experiences and support needs of male carers. This team provided support to, and engaged with, carers across the age spectrum. As noted by the team manager, "I think our youngest would be in his twenties, he's a brother actually, and the oldest would be a grandfather." I was given contact details for this young man and managed to speak to him twice to ask him to participate in the study but was not able to secure an interview. On one occasion, having agreed a date and time for an interview and arrived at the address provided, I discovered for a second time that he was not there. Observations noted in my fieldwork diary about why he was harder to pin down indicated something of the substantive character of his family life and the issues it presented for him:

Following two unanswered texts to remind him about the interview, I give him a call. It transpires that he isn't at home and can't be interviewed because his younger brother, who he is Special Guardian for and is 14, had stolen £500 from his account that morning. He was on the way to the bank to cancel his bankcard and to find out what he needs to do to recover the funds. He asks me in despair 'What do I do? Do I call the police on my own brother?'

Given the evident distress the participant conveyed, I decided not to pursue an interview. I deemed it unethical to burden him about participating in the research when his family priorities were so evidently pressing and of paramount importance. Despite my being unable to interview this young man, his case was nevertheless informative in terms of revealing some of the complexities and pressures that men were navigating and managing so that they could sustain their families.

The kinship care team manager also reflected on the team's continued engagements with several other family carers. The expectation from the local authority that men would put themselves forward to be caregivers was striking in this discussion, representing a potential barrier for men and suggesting less understanding about the marginalisations and constraints men may experience as prospective and actual caregivers. While the team were making a determined effort to create a community of carers via annual open days and festivals, these were not readily attended, especially by male carers. Sam, a kinship carer and one of the study participants, later commented that these events were a nice idea but what he really needed was some respite and adequate financing to support his grandson in the longer term.

Another issue observed was how difficult the service was finding it to sustain men's commitments to becoming carers even when they had been deemed a viable placement option. Referring to a recent case, the informant said:

> 'We've always had male carers, it's finding – it's taking the opportunity when the male carer has put himself forward. For example, just today, I was chasing up a grandfather who put himself forward to care for his granddaughter. We'd done a viability assessment which said he was going to need a full kinship assessment and he's come back today and said on reflection he feels other family members are better placed to care for this child. He hasn't illuminated anymore how that might be, which is a little disappointing … I think he realised that he as a single male carer living in another country, he was isolated … and isolating the child from her birth family.'

While it was difficult for the team to extrapolate the reasons for his withdrawal, in this case the carer had expressed legitimate concerns, as a single man living in another country, about isolating the child. Despite this participant's expression of disappointment, it was clear that there was limited capacity or resource available to the team to explore the full extent of the reasons behind this withdrawal and how or whether the outcome might be changed. Nevertheless, this interview offered rich insights into the local support context and some of the policy mechanisms and assumptions that might contribute to men being absented from opportunities that might enable them to be formally recognised as carers. As noted, men are there and they are present in family and service contexts but they are rendered less visible because opportunities to engage them are limited by time and resources.

Following this interview, a list of contacts for eight men was offered. While two were unreachable, the rest participated in the research and this proved to be one of the more fruitful avenues for identifying men to participate.

Voluntary and third sector agencies

Individual semi-structured interviews were also conducted with managers and support workers from local voluntary and third sector agencies. They included a support worker for a faith-based charity supporting the rehabilitation of ex-offenders, a manager of a kinship care support charity and the chief executive officers (CEOs) of two charities, one providing dedicated support to carers in the city and the other providing youth services alongside intensive family support to parents and grandparents for families affected by alcohol or drugs. These interviews revealed more general issues about the gendered nature of service support in the city and how these might be addressed, as well as detailed accounts of the men they were supporting and the kinds of complex issues that they were navigating.

The CEO for the charity that was supporting carers confirmed the problem of the gendered nature of the support landscape identified in existing research. Reflecting on the local offer in the city and some of the challenges presented, she explained that "there is a massive gap in needs, recognition and identification for male carers. Some of the key issues we face in engaging men include that men can be hard to engage, they might not want support and resources are very tight." During the interview she explained that she had tried to improve the accessibility of the service for men by addressing the issue of having a majority female workforce in her organisation by hiring two male workers, although there is limited evidence to suggest that the gender of workers is essential to effective support for men (Scourfield et al,

2014). Caring and compassionate support is often valued much more highly by men than working with a male worker (Robb et al, 2015). For this organisation, the issue of identifying men who specifically identified themselves as carers remained a key concern. There is a distinct parallel here with the kinship care identity. Many grandparents and family members who engage in informal kinship care are unfamiliar with the term kinship care, for example, until they experience formal state intervention and are required to identify themselves in this way to secure resources for their families.

The CEO also elaborated some useful observations on the different kinds of caring responsibilities that men had in different socioeconomic contexts and localities in the city. She explained that in wealthier areas of the city the charity was more likely to support elderly male carers who were looking after their wives and partners. Reflecting patterns of health inequality across the city as well as the national picture, men in these areas statistically live longer than those residing in lower socioeconomic areas and are therefore more likely to become carers. There is evidence that the gendered landscape of care is changing in older age, both nationally and internationally. In the UK, 15.1% of the population aged 65 years and over are male spousal carers, as compared to 13.5% who are women (Milligan and Morbey, 2016). Confirming observations made by the other professionals who were interviewed, the CEO also noted that those living in low-income areas of the city were more likely to be juggling multiple care responsibilities both for their own parents and children, with their own complex needs. Based on her experience of supporting carers and seeking to develop and proactively improve the support offer for men in the city, she outlined a useful framework comprising four key areas, summarised here, that require consideration by professionals:

- *Identification*: male carers need support to identify themselves as carers, and for appropriate support to be available when caring impacts on their lives.
- *Needs*: this is about thinking about how to help men but also manage their expectations in a context of limited flexibility,
- *Family dynamics*: this influences the extent of stress and anxiety faced but may also still contribute to the loneliness and isolation male carers may experience.
- *Men's physical and mental well-being*: men are likely to face specific physical and mental health challenges. In terms of mental health, countering traditional ideas about gender and masculinity is important.

Mirroring findings by Emmel et al (2007), it was the individuals carrying out fringe work in low-income localities who had long-standing and trusting relationships with individuals and families in the locality. Through reflection on their own practice, these professionals provided insights about how to actualise the four components described above in their everyday approaches. In the MPLC study, these professionals demonstrated a keen awareness of the problems male carers were facing and were actively tailoring their offer to the needs of the men they were supporting. More detailed discussions in the interviews about the men they were supporting demonstrated just how complex and extensive were the issues that some men in low-income families were facing. Support was tailored to concerns as wide ranging as (grand)parenting, relationships and communication issues, and guidance around legal issues and mental health. Depending on the age of the men they were supporting, some services were also offering practical help in relation to education, employment, housing and finances.

The effects of a complex set of legal and policy processes and austerity-driven changes were also in evidence that, in some cases, were mitigating against men's efforts to be involved in their children's lives. A support worker for a faith-based charity outlined several challenging cases of men he was working with who were seeking to be more involved as fathers, which required them to navigate a complex range of personal issues and complicated systems. In one account of a 40-year-old father who had limited mental capacity but wanted to be more involved in the lives of his four children, the support worker described the intensive support he needed to provide to help him to traverse the changing legal system.

> 'When I first started dealing with this case, he'd go to one of these solicitors over the road and they'd be like, "Right, sign that," and the state would pay the Legal Aid to do this. That's not going to happen anymore.[1] He's got to represent himself. I've got a letter that says he needs a litigation friend at any court appearance. He can't understand sophisticated court processes in any sense.
>
> 'So we've had to do quite a bit of learning around this, because I don't want to say that he can be [involved as a dad], it's not my decision, that's for the courts, but I do want him to get a fair crack at it and he's asked for that support. So we've first of all supported him to get to the doctor's to get his medication set up, make sure his house is all right, and then a couple of weeks ago we had to get

a stack of forms like that [indicates a large pile], C100s[2] they're called, and fill them all in.'

Several of the professionals interviewed were critical and reflexive about the impacts of welfare, employment and family policy changes at the time and aware of the effects of the structural inequalities that were impacting on the lives of the men they were supporting. The CEO of the large charity supporting men with complex needs described their attempts to identify and respond to high rates of suicide in one ward in the city (examined from the perspectives of residents and participants in Chapter 7). This organisation, working in collaboration with a community centre in another low-income ward of the city, was doing important work to manufacture and scaffold community-based supports and engagements among men with limited financial resources to tackle their isolation:

> 'We've also done quite specialist work around better communication ... bringing them [men] together to look at how they can support each other and relate to one another. Only to find that three-quarters of them are now in employment, not drinking, and their lives have turned around because someone has cared about them, bringing them to a safe space, and actually got them to talk about their anxieties. So, we generally find in our experience that men aren't listened to and the avenues for them to go to are quite limited.'

The significance of specific support for men's anxieties and mental health was a major emergent theme and something that Don (a pseudonym) reflected on. Don was one of the main gatekeepers for the IGE study, who also agreed to support the MPLC research. As a manager for a local charity providing extensive support to kinship carers, he noted the need for a new support group specifically for men that would focus on what he referred to as their 'internal violence', namely, the mental and physical health effects on men caused by keeping problems bottled up and not dealing with them. The expectation that men should maintain emotional control and that they are rational and responsible at times of distress, particularly in public, is linked to more traditional models of masculinity and is a stereotype that is starting to be disrupted within community-based support groups (for example, Simpson and Richards 2019). Don was an astute observer of the processes that he thought were absenting men from family contexts, especially where the state intervenes. Contrary to popular belief, he suggested that it is not difficult to encourage male carers and grandfathers to attend support groups. Challenging wider assumptions that men are hard to reach (Neale and Davies, 2015) and to get talking, he explained that they are most likely to open up and communicate when they attend. However, he suggested that they are less likely to do so if their wives are present. His observation was that the presence of their wives often changed support dynamics, influencing what men were likely to say.

Reflecting on the diverse families he was working with, Don also discussed some of the possible issues grandfathers as kinship carers might face. Based on work he was doing with four grandfathers who were kinship carers at the time of the interview, he suggested that men are especially vulnerable to accusations of being abusive to daughters (including in-laws) and female children and that accusations of this kind, whether true or not, can have negative implications for men's familial and personal relationships. He noted that once wives and sons have doubt in their minds, this can be highly disruptive to their familial relationships in the longer term. Lending weight to his observations, three of the MPLC participants later identified this as a concern with little prompting. These were mid-life father Will, age 44, and kinship carers Reggie and Dougie. In-depth analyses of their cases are developed further in Chapters 5 (Dougie and Reggie) and 7 (Will).

Don was careful to say that such issues are not specific to low-income families, but affected kinship care families more generally. Kinship care can be especially risky for men, especially when gendered assumptions and the sexualisation of young people combine and affect what are ostensibly private, yet highly regulated, family contexts. Similar concerns about risks to men in kinship care were also expressed by a female participant in a study of kinship carers seeking advice and support from a national advice and advocacy telephone support line (Tarrant et al, 2017). In this study, a grandmother explained that she had decided not to pursue a Special Guardianship Order[3] so that she could protect her husband. Her grandchildren had accused their father of abusing them and she expressed legitimate concerns that they might do the same to her husband.

Don also highlighted a range of issues and disadvantages that kinship families are required to manage, often without support or training, including care for grandchildren with learning disabilities and/or Foetal Alcohol Syndrome, which can cause acute behavioural problems in children. He also noted the challenges of managing often toxic relationships with parents and children in contact centres, which, he suggested, are in buildings that have become increasing worn down and shabby under the increasing pressures of austerity-driven funding cuts. These latter issues were not specific to the participants in the MPLC study but provided important contextual insight into the complexity of the lives of these families and the kinds of support needs and requirements that services may need to be aware of. Don's insights were further revealing of the processes through which men might be required to become active family participants and how they might be affected by evolving and often messy patterns of need and dependency in these family contexts.

Overall, Don was a busy and energetic character and often difficult to pin down. He was unable to provide specific contacts for participants, but he did invite me to attend one of the support groups for kinship carers while it was still running. I was able to recruit two participants via this approach: Dougie and Reggie. Don also attended the knowledge-exchange workshop, to which the chapter now turns.

Knowledge-exchange workshop

Reflecting the participatory ethos underpinning the study, a knowledge-exchange workshop was held with professionals from third sector organisations based in the city to complement and enhance the insights emerging from the interviews. This was attended by five professionals, all of whom had shown an interest in the study and had contributed to insights either in interviews and/or via consultation prior to the workshop. The third sector in the city comprises a range of voluntary organisations, charities, community groups, informal self-help groups and community work by faith groups. There are also identifiable services providing support to families living on a low income, some of which are targeted specifically at men or that support men to tackle key issues that may affect their lives. The participants in the workshop were representatives from three local charities, a dads' group and a housing association. The group therefore comprised individuals and organisations providing support for men of all ages across the city. Specifically, the participants included a housing support manager with expertise in local housing and welfare policy; Don, the manager of the charity supporting grandparents and other family members who are kinship carers; a young dads' support group coordinator for a group located in a low-income ward of the city; an organiser of an urban walking group to support men with their mental health; and a manager for a new charity supporting older adult men experiencing multiple disadvantages. The meeting had a three-fold aim, including (1) to test out some of the emerging substantive findings from the existing data that was analysed in the early phase of MPLC (presented to and discussed with the participants in the session, see Appendix 2); (2) to further explore what evidence gaps there might be about men and their support needs; and (3) to consider what evidence might be produced to inform existing support provision in the city.

The discussions informed the MPLC research in line with local priorities and ensured that it was rooted in men's real concerns and life experiences in low-income localities (Tarrant, 2015). Complementing the interview data, additional reflections about what these participants were observing as key issues for men and boys in low-income families and localities were also captured.

The discussions at the workshop were structured around a number of activities, including a round of introductions to each individual and invited reflections about why they were interested in the research; a stakeholder analysis exercise of the local policy and support context; reflections on the early emerging findings from previous research to prompt discussions about men living on a low income and the current experiences and priorities of the third sector in the city; and group reflections on the proposed research questions and their appropriateness for generating relevant evidence for the third sector in the city. These discussions confirmed that the MPLC research questions were valuable, highlighted additional areas for the research to explore and strengthened the case for researching the lives, experiences and support needs of men in different generational positions.

In the introductory statements made by the attendees of the meeting, it became clear that there was a commitment by the local third sector to engage men and to address their needs, no matter how complex. Community groups were described as positive sources of care and community for men and were deemed the most effective way of tackling the social isolation that many men report whether they are embedded in families or not. A common observation of the group was that, regardless of the care responsibilities men may have or of their age or generational position, under current social and economic conditions men are highly likely to become socially isolated. They described a complex set of factors driving men's social isolation in low-income contexts, as illustrated in this excerpt of the conversation:

Young dads' worker: When you move into adulthood and you move into being a father, you can often lose that social aspect, whether it's through economic terms, like looking at here in terms of how poverty affects lives, but from going and being in a social group at school or just after school, that can just dissolve. So I think it's [referring to tailored support for men] something that does have a real value and if there can be an educational aspect to it, and if there can be a progressive aspect to it, then it's all the better.

Housing and welfare manager: We come across a lot of men who are very isolated. But if you do give them the opportunity and the mechanism to join a group they really enjoy that social interaction and really respond to that kind of social interaction, which perhaps then brings them into contact with more mainstream services ... I mean, our advice service was just inundated. And the problems they were bringing to us were complex and multiple, lots of issues. I'm always going to come back to poverty and welfare reform to some extent, but people trying to cope with changes to council tax support, the under-occupancy, because [city council] have had a policy of placing single men in multi-storey properties ... not seeing the bedroom tax on the horizon.

Urban walk organiser: They'll go and jump off.

Manager of charity for men with complex needs: The flip side – that man desert thing [terminology used in the Fractured Families family report at the start of this book] – just strikes me as being really weird, it doesn't really resonate, the man desert issue, but I certainly know that other places I've lived in the past, there's been a policy about putting single-parent families onto an estate. And that will have created some of that, but I thought that would have gone out of fashion some decades ago.

In these accounts, social isolation is described as the key factor in bringing men to services. As the young dads' worker observes, community-based support that is progressive in its outlook and that offers new skills can play a vital role in tackling men's isolation. Community-based services also act as an important bridge between communities and mainstream services. The group theorised that men's experiences of isolation are attributable to a complex mix of structural inequalities and factors, including their increasingly insecure attachments to the labour market, limited and decreasing welfare support, caring for a child or family member as a single parent or carer, being single and living without family, living in poverty and insecure housing and having increasingly limited community-based supports. Local housing policy changes were also observed as significant, as well as increasingly insecure transitions to adulthood and fatherhood, unstable relationships with female partners and the mothers of their children and financial insecurity. For young men, the erosion of educational opportunities, poverty, gendered expectations, such as being a provider, and policy change are also paramount. The housing and welfare manager, for example, noted:

> 'The thing with young people as well, the thing about fatherhood, we are often going through both the young women and the young men as well, and it's this sense of – a real sense of excitement, the same as any of us would have felt having a child. It's almost like this is a blank page, this is a really good start. But the stress then of having a newborn baby when you're a young person but more crucially you're in poverty just taints the whole experience to such an extent that it's a wonder that any of them get through it.'

She further reflected on the stigma young men experience in the context of limited educational and employment opportunities, making direct connections to experiences of poverty that in the past have been found to slip out of sight where services focus instead on individual drug or alcohol problems or on 'individual attitudes, values and priorities' (Featherstone et al, 2017: 105):

> 'One of the things I find is people, often they will mistake a lack of education for a lack of intelligence. It's so offensive. And it's about opportunities that are available ... what I see from our core work, which is with young men, is the lack of opportunity. And that's just getting worse. And yet they're born into this narrative of being required to be this great provider and to have this great job. And I just don't see those great jobs that are actually open to the young people that I'm working with. And they get so frustrated, who wouldn't? And so the stress that that then invokes and the stress that is involved in poverty.'

The charity CEO noted: "It either comes out as stress, frustration, anger, or it becomes the other way, despair and a kind of inertia."

Issues like these were addressed specifically by the community group for fathers, which provided comprehensive support for young men to come together as parents. This group also offered support to young men in other aspects of their lives, including helping them to search for employment, to complete legal documents and forms to secure welfare, and support to develop a range of life skills, like DIY, cookery, gardening and arts-based activities.

Group-based activities like these, that bring young men together around their shared identities as fathers, are proven to help to address the isolation and loneliness many young men experience (Hanna, 2018). Don observed a similar set of issues experienced by the older men he was supporting, which they expressed as stress, frustration and anger. However, what was distinctive for these men was that becoming a kinship carer much later in life was a key barrier to men's social participation. Don was especially proactive in the city in establishing support groups for grandparents to help to reduce the social isolation of kinship carers and provide a space for airing traumatic experiences within an experienced community. He noted the pressing need to create support opportunities that enable men to develop healthier relationships and express themselves to avoid anger and violence (Tarrant, 2015). Despite his ambitions for establishing more targeted support for male kinship carers around their mental health, towards the end of the study, the charity Don worked for was merged with a national charity due to funding constraints. Don, who was a single father himself, was compelled to retire early and so left the area. The support network, which was a vital lifeline for kinship carers and their families, ended without a viable replacement, although new support groups have since been established, funded by the third sector.

With regard to service provision for men with complex needs, it was argued that good support is about providing advice, advocating for men and assisting them in an informed way. Engagement with men with their own lived experiences and histories of complex social problems was also considered helpful. The support worker for men with complex needs said:

> 'We use people with lived experience as part of the project and part of the workforce on the project as well. And certainly when it comes to working with people who are particularly entrenched or outside the system, then it's

their ability to engage, it's not me … when they've seen somebody who's been through and is coming out the other side … it's powerful.'

It was acknowledged that services often find it difficult to engage men, and certainly, recent research about young fatherhoods turns the otherwise taken-for-granted assumption that men are hard to reach on its head, suggesting that often services are 'hard-to-access' (Neale et al, 2015). However, the professionals noted that men can be found in communal and community-based spaces like pubs and in betting shops and, with persistence they can and do engage in the longer term. It was apparent that the most effective services provide a safe environment for men and focus on working with and alongside them, rather than in a formal, head-on fashion.

Concluding remarks

The professional insights presented in this chapter confirm when and how men are present in family and service contexts. Men become most visible to services either when they are experiencing significant personal troubles themselves or when they are trying to secure resources and/or support on behalf of themselves or their families. The findings suggest that low-income families remain dependent on the third sector and services, which have a key role to play in providing support to families experiencing hardship. While there is evidence of the requirement for extensive resource and emotional exchange within and across households in low-income contexts for the purposes of survival (Emmel and Hughes, 2010), interventions and support provided by services remain essential for tackling isolation, signposting to mainstream services and engaging men as potential carers. The observations presented here provide some initial insights about how men's caring responsibilities and family participation in low-income contexts are shaped in a complex landscape of policy, employment, housing and legal requirements and processes. It is especially clear that when professionals and services are responsive to men, not only as parents and as family members but also to the complex and wide-ranging needs men may experience, then they are also better able to provide the intensive support that is sometimes required. These professionals were able to identify, understand and ensure support in relation to a much wider set of social determinants that affect men's lives, including employment and education, mental health concerns and social isolation, because they were attuned to the challenges and constraints of the contexts through which these problems were produced.

However, services may sometimes lack the resources and capacity to engage with men, even when they become visible to them. Those that do engage men reach them in all sorts of creative and often indirect ways that do not necessarily lend themselves readily as family support. Significantly, those that work with a compassionate and supportive ethos and with an understanding, rather than punitive, approach towards the varied needs of men, appear better able to support individual men and their families.

5

Men's caring arrangements and family trajectories

This chapter is the first of three that present analyses of men's accounts of their family participation and care trajectories. It explores the questions of how and in which ways men participate in their families in low-income contexts and foregrounds their diverse caring arrangements and family configurations and trajectories. An in-depth examination is presented of the diverse and divergent sets of caring arrangements described by men in different generational positions, drawing on empirical examples across the cases. The findings in this chapter demonstrate how caring arrangements in low-income families are both negotiated and contested over time. This includes across familial generations, between men and women and often in engagements with services and agencies external to families. Attention to these caring arrangements reveals how gendered and classed inequalities are reproduced within family practices, personal relationships and intergenerationally, sometimes requiring men to reassert their right to their families.

The dynamic processes and family trajectories of both the participants and their family members, which determined how the men's caring arrangements came to be, are also explored. Such processes are revealing of the social and relational character of men's caring arrangements in low-income contexts and of the circumstances and personal biographies that required these men to respond to and meet the support needs of their younger family members. Consideration of how the participants narrate their care responsibilities, caring masculinities and the family structures that produce them renders visible the diverse, relational pathways that characterise men's family participation in low-income family contexts across the lifecourse.

The vulnerable family contexts and caregiving arrangements that men manage and negotiate in low-income families also foreground often ignored forms of socially marginalised fatherhoods. These also happen to be fatherhoods that occur in contexts where men's ability to balance their earning capacities with family care are perhaps most subject to compromise or challenge (see O'Brien, 2011). Here, the often hidden and untapped potential of men's family participation in low-income contexts gains precedence.

Diverse caring arrangements

Reflecting the complexity and diversity of contemporary family forms and biographies, MPLC uncovered a varied set of caring arrangements and family configurations. Many of the family configurations described by the participants have been conceptualised as being those most likely to increase vulnerability to poverty (for example, Kelly and Daly, 2015; Mynarska et al, 2015; see also Chapter 3; Appendix 1). The family configurations the participants described included families headed by young parents, lone-parent families, families where someone (either a parent or/and child) has a disability, families with child protection concerns and kinship care families. The household circumstances of the participants were also diverse. Seven of the men had primary responsibilities for children and were lone parents, mostly following divorce or separation (typically the more-resourced men in their mid- to later life). One of these men was severely disabled and was occasionally cared for by his own child, and two were lone fathers caring for adult disabled sons. Seven were primary caregivers and were seeking or had secured kinship care status.[1] Eleven were non-resident, with limited access to their children (typically the younger men in the sample and those who were most deprived and frequented the community centre for social support, see Chapter 7), and one was a grandfather with a history of family poverty.

Even across this relatively small set of cases the family participation of these men was also incredibly varied and reflected a continuum of involvement in terms of contact with children. The lone fathers and kinship carers typically described more extensive engagement with the children they were responsible for and it is these men's cases, of the 26, that are predominantly considered here. The younger fathers and those in the most deprived circumstances described greater precarity and associated concerns that meant that they had a less regular or intensive presence in the lives of their children. For those who were primary caregivers to young children, their experiences were even more unusual. To make sense of this plethora of arrangements and divergent family trajectories, and to shed light on these men's family practices and responsibilities, I differentiate in this chapter between men in different generational positions. Each section therefore examines the experiences of families headed by young fathers, lone, mid-life fathers and kinship care families (although there was some slippage among categories as some of the young fathers were also lone fathers). The diversity of household arrangements, including non-residence, is also explored within these groupings.

Young fathers

Eight of the participants interviewed for MPLC were young fathers, which in policy terms refers to young men who experience a first pregnancy or have a child or children when they are aged 25 and under (Fatherhood Institute, 2013). These young men are most associated with the absent father discourses discussed in Chapter 1 and are often constructed as a problem in social policy (Duncan, 2010; Beggs Weber, 2012; Neale et al, 2015). As observed by the service providers in Chapter 4, these young men were experiencing especially precarious employment trajectories, linked to the insecure employment opportunities of their localities and to their own, often chaotic, family backgrounds. The extent of their precarity was also reflected by their dependencies on third sector and statutory services (see access pathway information in Table 5.1). Table 5.1

Table 5.1: The young fathers

Father	Age	Access pathway	Relationship status	Care status/residence
Adrian	18	Sheltered accommodation service	Not in relationship with MOC	Non-resident but weekly contact
Ashley	22	Housing association	Partnered (although relationship broken down in Wave 2)	Step-father in Wave 1; resident uncle Wave 2
Connor	16	Specialist education support team	Not in relationship with MOC, in a relationship	Non-resident to child (with questions over paternity)
Damien	14	Specialist education support team	In a relationship with MOC	Non-resident but weekly contact with child
Joe	22	Sheltered accommodation service	On/off relationship with MOC of second child	Non-resident to two children, with irregular contact
Reece	22	Re-accessed via specialist education support team and from Following Young Fathers study	Re-partnered	Non-resident to first child; resident with new partner who was due a baby
Ricky	22	Local support group for fathers	Single	Lone father
Shane[2]	27	Kinship care team	Partnered	Lone father

provides brief socio-demographic details of the young fathers including their age, current relationships status with the mother of their child(ren) (MOC), and their care and residence status with their children.

Like many of the young fathers interviewed for FYF (Neale et al, 2015), one of the baseline studies for MPLC, these participants expressed a desire to 'be there' for their children. However, a range of factors either mitigated against or enabled them to fulfil their expressed intentions. They therefore narrated an orientation towards caregiving, although practical circumstances and relationships with the mothers of children who acted as gatekeepers (Reeves et al, 2009; Neale and Patrick, 2016) were important in these processes, especially when they were the primary caregivers. The caring arrangements of the young fathers reflected a mixed picture ranging from non-residence to more unusual levels of fatherly caregiving where they were lone fathers and/or primary caregivers. These status were contingent on the marginalisations that are often experienced by young fathers residing in low-income families or localities. These include any combination of poverty; limited support in education, training or employment; unstable homes; volatile family backgrounds and periods in care; mental health issues; and experiences of offending and domestic violence (as both victims and perpetrators). The processes leading to these arrangements, as well as how they are experienced by these young men and their families are explored next.

Lone-father caring arrangements

Two of the young dads described care processes where they actively fought for parental responsibility for their children via legal processes. These transitions to secure primary paternal responsibility required navigation through complex social care and legal systems. For both Ricky and Shane, their journeys to becoming primary caregivers for their children were fraught with challenge. Accessing help via a fathers' support group, Ricky was a lone parent caring for four-year-old daughter Tia.[3] The interview took place at his new home, which he had recently secured through the council. He explained that he could no longer live with his mum, who lived down the road. Her house was already over-occupied because she was looking after his 15-year-old brother and informally providing kinship care to two of her grandchildren, a common experience in low-income communities (Hughes and Emmel, 2011). Ricky also occasionally babysat for them to support his mum. He explained that while Tia was the result of a planned pregnancy, he had been depressed when he first met her mother and had not really wanted to be in a relationship with her. He explained that, following Tia's birth, her mother referred to her simply as 'it'. She eventually withdrew as a parent and Tia was placed with a foster carer. Ricky decided to fight for primary parental responsibility for her through the courts, which caused him a great deal of distress:

> 'Her mum just walked away from her. She did see her for one night but didn't bath her, didn't feed her. And then couple of weeks after I said to my foster carers can I move in with her? And the foster carers said they don't know. We'll ask the social workers. And she said yeah. And I moved in for three months – because it was like a mothers and baby unit, but it was their first time going to be a father and baby unit ... Went through all the court and now I've had her now ... my foster carer seen me upset, usually sees me like happy. But this one got me really badly.'

Significantly, the support of the foster carers and the responsiveness of both the social workers and the courts played a key role in enabling Ricky to acquire responsibility for his daughter, although Ricky was unable to explain why he had not been considered as a placement option in the first place. While he noticeably experienced the mother and baby unit as gendered, the support of social services was essential for enabling him to be recognised as Tia's primary care giver. However, they did not approach him as a possible placement option. Ricky had to put himself forward before he was considered.

Shane also went through court processes to become a primary caregiver to Brittany (age 10) and Harrison (age 8). His experience was different to Ricky's in that he received a letter unexpectedly, informing him that he might be the biological father of two children in care who were about to be adopted. Their mother was struggling to cope with the care of her four other children and she suspected that he was their biological father (she had six children in total). Aged 24 at the time, Shane was given just seven days by the courts to prove his paternity. A DNA test confirmed that he was Harrison's biological father, but not the father of Harrison's half-sister Brittany. Shane determined that it would be better to keep the children together, saying he 'couldn't have split them up'. He was approached by the Kinship Care team and awarded paternal responsibility for his biological son and a Special Guardian Order for Brittany. He spent eight months visiting the children fortnightly to get to know them, which increased to weekly visits and then a sleep-over a week before they began to live with him.

When Shane first took on the children's care he was still living with his mother but he was later able to negotiate social housing for himself and the children. In both Shane and Ricky's cases, the ability to acquire social housing was essential to providing a stable and secure home for them and their children and a clear trajectory towards greater independence, prompted by and incorporating familial care. However, this process took time, and Shane required support from services because he needed a three-bedroomed house by law to accommodate both children. In UK legislation, male and female siblings cannot share a bedroom because of their gender and the legalities around 'looked after' children. Shane explained that despite being responsible for two care-experienced children he was charged incorrectly for the bedroom tax, one of the more contentious of the UK government's austerity policies, and was forced to renegotiate it with the council. Shane also described some of the early interpersonal problems he negotiated with Brittany when she first moved in with him, including how he managed her early resistance to his paternal role:

> ' "You're not my dad" and this, that and the other and I just said, "Look, I'm not biologically your father darling, but I'm your dad. I'm looking after you, I'm always going to be here for you." We had a couple of spats like that, but I think she's got her head around it now. She understands that she's mine and this is her forever home.'

He also explained that his biological son, five-year-old Harrison, continued to have complex behavioural issues, including bed wetting and breaking toys, although he was not convinced this was related to his son's past neglect as was suggested by the social worker. Shane continues to allow the children to see their mum and half-siblings and they have an amicable relationship.

The financial arrangements for the children were also complicated and he explained that he sometimes went without food to ensure the children never went hungry. He left employment to settle the children and the financial entitlements are both complex to manage and inadequate. He explained that while he is entitled to child benefit and child tax credits for Harrison, he cannot claim the same financial support for Harrison as he can for Brittany. Some of the finances received for the care of Harrison are therefore deducted from Brittany's maintenance allowance. Despite these difficulties, Shane was good humoured about his circumstances and had no regrets about changing his life to support his children:

> 'Obviously, it's hard work being a single parent, but I just thought it can't be that bad, just get it done! I'm one of those people who just gets something done rather than moaning

and bitching about it. I will just get it done and then cry myself to sleep at night! ... I'm only joking! [Laughs]'

Despite describing himself as a single parent in this extract, Shane also discussed a new relationship he had established with a woman who also has her own young son. Reflecting the dynamic nature of family vulnerability and change, he explained that he was hopeful for the future of this relationship and that he valued the additional support it offered. As lone fathers, Ricky and Shane do not conform to wider assumptions that young fathers are dependents in family contexts, demonstrating instead how they fulfil their responsibilities to their children in contexts of great adversity and financial hardship. They do this even though the processes of gaining primary care responsibility are messy, tenuous and dependent on the positive involvements of courts and other agencies.

Social fathering and wider familial care practices

Caregiving for wider family members and those in local support networks was identified among the young fathers and grandfathers in the IGE and FYF studies (see Appendix B) and emerged as significant in MPLC too. Ashley, whom his sister Kara and his partner Jess affectionately call 'Nanny McAsh', had perhaps the most unusual care situation relative to the rest of the young fathers interviewed. Ashley was recruited to MPLC via a local housing association. His biography reflects a chaotic history of deprivation, characterised by volatile family relationships with both his biological and adoptive parents that resulted in time spent in a children's home and enforced separation from his siblings. Following his time in the children's home, he became involved in the informal economy, selling cannabis and cocaine, for which he was caught and spent six weeks in prison. Ashley, who explained how his early experiences have made him depressed, has been supported into secure housing via the local housing association and into employment. At the time of the first interview he was working, albeit in a fund-raising job that he disliked, not least because it was exploitative.

Ashley was interviewed twice and, while he was recommended to the study, it became apparent in the first interview that he was not a biological father. However, he was providing care to two-year-old Caid, the son of Jess, his girlfriend of five months, whom he says he loves as his own. Caid's father was domestically violent to Ashley's partner and they described him simply as a 'sperm donor'. This first interview became an unexpected family focus group (Brown, 2015), as both Ashley's sister and girlfriend were present for the discussions. Caid was also present, as was Ashley's nephew, a small baby sitting in a bouncer at the edge of the room. The participants described the strong bond that Ashley has with Caid, as well as the strong ethic of care that they express for one another as a family:

Kara:	He's [Caid] got more of a bond with Ashley than he has with any other man.
Ashley:	They're energetic, aren't they? I'm energetic. I've got loads of energy to get rid of.
Jess:	It gives us a break as well. Like me and Ashley will look after Caid to give Kara a break from it all so she has her own time and stuff. So like Ashley will take Caid out for the day, gives me a break from Caid as well. So we all help each other out really.

These narratives are revealing of how embedded and present Ashley is in his family context, which, contrasted with his family history, is much more stable and enables opportunities for reciprocity among family members. Alternative practices of care were in evidence among men and families even in some of the most precarious local contexts. Particularly striking in the narratives of Ashley and these young women were the everyday practices of care that emerge in localities, especially in austerity contexts (Power and Hall, 2017; Bonner-Thomson and McDowell, 2020). These often unnoticed yet essential practices comprise the complex social infrastructures and tapestries of care (Hall, 2019) that are crucial to the fabric of everyday life on a low income. Such practices maintain horizontal ties and social bonds among family, friends and neighbours and are an invisible form of participation. In the following exchange, they reflected:

Ashley:	We all look after everyone. We'll knock on each other's door and go, 'Have you got any sugar? Have you got any coffee? Got any milk?'
Jess:	Doing my weekly shop at Aldi. Don't need to go to Sainsbury's. Got this? Got that? I think offer them money for something that I need or something. Like I'll be cooking a chilli round here and I'll forget that I need an onion. And I'll go round and ask for an onion or I'll give you some money for an onion. Like no, just take the onion.
Kara:	It's an onion.

Jess: But still, like most grocers, it's like a quid for three onions. You know what I mean? That's a lot of money.

Low-income families often engage in processes of mutual support and exchange with one another and others in their localities as a strategy of survival that enables them to meet their everyday needs, and it was no different for this family. Interestingly, when I returned to meet Ashley for a second interview, having completed the photovoice task, he was no longer in a relationship with Jess, who, he explained had returned to a relationship with Caid's biological father. His claims to fatherhood had therefore changed. However, he remained close to his sister and highly involved in the care of his nephew, who featured heavily in the images taken.

Non-resident arrangements

Like Ashley, not all of the young fathers were able to sustain access to their children following the breakdown of their relationships, reporting sporadic or even lost access. Connor, aged 16, described a challenging set of processes that, despite his best efforts to remain involved, eventually led to a loss of access to his son altogether. At the time his son was born he was 15 years old and was dealing with anger issues linked to the pressures of education, the divorce of his parents, the stigma associated with becoming a young father, the breakdown of his relationship with the mother of his son after she 'cheated' on him and questions about his paternity. He explained:

> 'I didn't know about the pregnancy until she was eight months gone and she came back to me and I was already with another girlfriend and I dearly loved her, really did love her, and erm, I couldn't leave her and we was having like a meeting type thing in her living room with some social workers and she was like "I really want to get back together and be a family" and I was like "I can't though because I won't love you the same". And then after that everything just seemed to be like, always need to be there on time to see my son, when I wasn't there she'd be really upset and she'd always try and force a relationship, which were very upsetting ...'

Connor struggled to forge workable routines and arrangements around social services and his ex-partner and it was difficult for him to sustain longer-term engagement with his child, especially while he remained unsure if the child was his.

Difficulties in sustaining relationships with children when non-resident were also linked to the housing insecurity experienced by young fathers. Adrian (age 18), who was also no longer in a relationship with the mother of his daughter (age 4) and only saw her every other weekend, described sofa surfing and staying with friends following the breakdown of his partnership with the mother of his daughter and related disagreements with his own parents. Living in a hostel at the time of the interview he said:

> 'I was with my daughter's mum. Obviously lived with her. Our relationship finished but before I moved in with her me and my parents were not on the best of terms. So I couldn't really go back there when I moved out of her house. That's why I'm living where I am now ... we already had our daughter. It was like last year now. We was together but I didn't live with her for that long. I lived with her for about a year. We broke up last year. Recently I've been kind of homeless. I just stayed with my cousins or friends. Just stay where I could until something got sorted. Wasn't that bad. I was just staying on sofas ... I was just chilling and wound up going to sleep on the sofa downstairs. It wasn't bad, I wasn't like living out in the streets. Could have been worse I guess.'

The precarity, homelessness and insecure housing trajectory described here reflected a shared experience among many of the young fathers in this research (see also Neale and Ladlow, 2015). According to Bonner-Thompson and McDowell (2020), sofa surfing and reliance on friends is a precarious but alternative form of caregiving that has increased among young people in the austerity context, but one that can have pernicious implications for father involvement, especially for young fathers. Contrasted with Ricky and Shane, who were able to secure social housing and remain involved with their children, Adrian was living a nomadic life and had no stable housing or familial base to enable him to develop a secure relationship with his child.

Reece and Joe had also lost access to their eldest children, but, as the eldest of the young fathers interviewed, both aged 22, they both had new partners with whom they had second children. Loss of access to their first child was because of tenuous or broken relationships with the mothers. The extent of complexity in the trajectories of deprivation that some of the young fathers were negotiating was articulated particularly clearly by Joe. Joe, 22 years old at the time of the interview, explained that he had two children by two different partners. His dad, who was violent to Joe's mum and her children, left home when Joe was 15 years old. Joe explained how, for a period of one year following his father's departure, he was expected to become "the man of the house" and looked after his younger siblings to support his mum. These pressures meant that his behaviour progressively worsened at this time and his mum "kicked him out" when he was 16 as she could no longer cope. He also linked his behavioural issues to his anger and to the friendships he made in his neighbourhood. He explained that he "went rogue" and spent time sofa surfing and staying with friends. Joe described a short stint in prison after leaving home, linked to alcohol misuse, perpetration of domestic violence and anger issues. He linked the negative aspects of his trajectory to his parents' break-up, which he found very difficult. In line with more traditional and normative expectations of masculinity, he also explained that his stepfather had advised him to lock these emotions away, advice that he now actively contests:

> 'I know I've got to get myself sorted before anything else. If I can't get myself sorted … I'm not saying I can't look after my little boys when I have them, but I can't look after them if I can't look after myself first. I need to put myself first. I always used to put everyone else in front of me.'

As evidence of his commitment to self-care, Joe was accessing drug and alcohol support for young people and was seeking counselling. Joe recognised the importance of self-care before he could look after his children properly and be fully involved as a father. Palpable in his narrative and despite having navigated a challenging transition to adulthood marked by poverty and deprivation, was a feeling of having lost his way and being unsure how he could balance his responsibilities for his children while also securing stable housing and employment and remaining responsible for his own well-being.

Lone, mid-life fatherhood

Four of the men who were not young fathers were lone fathers with primary care responsibilities for their children (Table 5.2). These men describe varied and complex pathways to father involvement as lone fathers. In contrast to the young fathers, whose pathways reflect greater precarity, these men describe care trajectories that have resulted in

Table 5.2: The lone fathers

Name	Age	Access pathway	Employment	Relationship status	Children	Disability
Joseph	45	Housing and welfare charity	Unemployed	Divorced	Two sons (both non-resident) Daughters (age 17 and 14, both resident)	Personally disabled
Matthew	55	Recruitment flyer at carers' support group	Unemployed, volunteer	Divorced and single	One son (age 30)	Adult son
Rory	61	Recruitment flyer at carers' support group	Unemployed, semi-retired	Divorced twice and not in a relationship	One son (age 30)	Adult son
Shaun	38	Charity supporting men with complex needs	Unemployed, volunteer	In a relationship (not MOC)	Daughters (age 3 and 6, both resident)	N/A

otherwise unusual parenting and care arrangements, albeit ones that were challenging to secure and difficult to sustain.

All were unemployed and described problems accessing secure, flexible employment because of their care responsibilities. All but Joseph, who was physically disabled, were active in their communities and engaged in voluntary activities. Notably, three of these men, Joseph, and Matthew and Rory who were caring for adult disabled sons, described experiences of disability within their families. The narratives of these three men are considered in this section (I say more about Shaun in Chapter 6) to illustrate some of the challenges that lone fathers experience and continue to navigate in order to remain involved as fathers. Families where one or more members are disabled are especially vulnerable to poverty, stigma and marginalisation (Mynarska et al, 2015). Their marginalisation is also replicated in academic research, where fathers are neglected in literatures that examine the experiences of parenting with disability or parenting a child with a disability. They are also rarely considered in policy, practice or organisational contexts.

Rory, aged 61 and Matthew, aged 55, were both lone parents. Both described histories of turbulent relationships with the mothers of their children, including difficult and expensive divorces. Rory, who had four children with his first wife, remarried and had his fifth child, a now adult son who has Asperger's syndrome and with whom he resides. His second divorce was also costly and problematic. He explains that his ex-wife initially refused to let him see his son, so he took her to court to secure shared residence. This cost him £4,000 which he had to get loans to pay for. He is angry that this did not cost his ex-wife anything. While he has friendships with other women, he explained that because his son is so reliant on him it makes it difficult to form other relationships. Rory is the named carer for his son and had been for six years at the time of interview. His son is highly dependent on him and will interact only with select people, including his paternal grandmother. When I asked Rory who his main responsibility was for, he said his son, and likened his role to employment:

'[Son's name], 24/7. It is a 24/7, 52-weeks-a-year job. There's no let-up. You don't get respite. People with certain conditions, yes, people can have like a week's respite. I know [respite centre name], they've got a respite centre there where people can go in for a week. I don't get that because [son] will not go there. He will let his grandma come and let me go for a few days, but … He knows that he can rely on me. He can rely on me for everything. He's secure with me. I'm reliable. His mother's not reliable. His sisters aren't reliable, his two sisters. He doesn't have anything to do with them.

'I don't get respite. Well, a lot of men and women are probably in the same boat as me. It's when they've got partners, yes, they can get a bit of respite, but because I'm on my own, I don't get it.'

The vulnerability Rory expressed here related to both his status as a lone parent and to a lack of opportunity for support and respite.

Despite having comparable family circumstances, Matthew expressed his own vulnerability as a lone father in terms of economic vulnerability (a theme that is subject to more in-depth analysis in Chapter 6). Describing an equally challenging and expensive divorce, he painted a picture of an intense period that required him to juggle childcare for his son with work. While his ex- mother-in-law initially helped with childcare for her grandson, she wanted to charge Matthew the same as a child minder would following the separation. The divorce process was therefore characterised by multiple vulnerabilities linked to his new status as a single carer; a lack of local, affordable childcare options; a problematic family support network in which he experienced a loss of power and agency, especially in his relationship with his ex-wife and her family; expensive legal processes; and employment inflexibility. Only his relatively stable employment history to this point meant that he did not experience the housing precarity that the young fathers discussed.

> 'I had no money, I had to haggle with my mum-in-law how much money. She wanted the same as a child minder. And I couldn't afford a child minder. So we haggled. I was going through a divorce. I had solicitors. My ex-wife got legal aid. You can't get it now. Even though she was living with this guy. They were managing a pub so no outgoings. They got legal aid and I didn't. When I was struggling, she never once let me off the money. Even when I was burgled. Came home and everything had gone. I had to cancel all my house insurance because I couldn't afford them. Solicitor's letters on the doorstep for the money. And they came up and she said "Have you got my money?" I had to borrow money off a friend to pay my mortgage that month and it's something I'll never forget.'

Matthew also described the emotional costs of his divorce which led to a period of depression after later being made redundant, and associated physical ill-health, in which he "walked around like a zombie" and "on both legs – they rapidly came up in red sores … it was just stress". At the time of interview Matthew was applying for jobs at local charities but was unsure if he would be able to do the hours, which were proving to be too inflexible for him around the support needs of his son.

As noted, Joseph was physically disabled himself. He was also a lone parent and not in a relationship. The parenting experiences of men who father with disabilities is a particular area of empirical neglect (Kilkey and Clarke, 2010; O'Brien, 2011). In a rare intervention Kilkey and Clarke (2010) demonstrated some important common experiences shared by men who father with a disability or impairment, as well as a diversity of circumstances. Drawing on two studies, one that included fathers with a disability in a parent-focused study and the other that focused specifically on fathering and disability, they found that these fathers may encounter specific difficulties with fulfilling the expectations of the breadwinner role and the need to adapt fathering practices and engagements with the mothers of their children, within the constraints that their physical and/or sensory impairments imposed. Their research also highlighted variation in terms of ethnicity, socioeconomic status, age, partner status and the timing of experience within the lifecourse. They also identified the need to further explore the intersections of fathering disability with other categories that tend to be problematised, including single, non-resident, older, unemployed and poor or socially excluded fathers.

Interviewed for the MPLC study, 45-year-old Joseph was a lone father with primary responsibility for his two daughters, aged 17 and 14. He had diabetes neuropathy, which had disabled him by affecting the nerve endings in his legs and resulted in his being workless. His two older children were non-resident; one was married and had a daughter and the other has learning difficulties and lives with his mother. Joseph was divorced and, following the break-up, his two youngest daughters had said that they wanted to live with their dad. They went to court and he got custody of his youngest daughter within eight weeks. His ex-wife accused him of brainwashing and blackmailing their daughters, something he strenuously denied. Despite being physically immobile and being cared for at times by his 14-year-old daughter, Joseph had been deemed fit for work at a work capability assessment. He was especially close to his own father, who was his main confidant, but when his father died Joseph became more socially isolated. This was the result of a combination of pressures including his divorce, his care responsibilities for two young daughters as a single father, unemployment, his disability and the loss of his father, all of which led to a period of alcohol dependency in an effort to cope. Because of his physical pain, Joseph relied on his daughters being self-sufficient and so emphasised the importance of teaching them how to be independent:

> 'It has made them start and have to do more things for themselves. With her being 12, rather than make her tea I'll say, "Right you get something and I'll help you do it" or "I'll tell you what, I'll do it and you do it", because they are skills they need to learn aren't they? At 12 years old, when I was a kid, I could cook and clean and do a lot of things.'

He later suggested that the requirement to find employment competed with his parenting responsibilities much more than his personal and physical challenges, a point I return to later.

Like the young fathers, the involvement of these men was fraught with tensions and required careful and costly navigation through complex legal systems. Despite the emotional and financial costs of lone fatherhood, these men invest heavily in the care of their (in some cases adult) children often in structural contexts that increase their vulnerabilities and mitigate against their intentions and abilities to provide care.

Older male carers and grandfathers

Older male kin carers and grandfathers are a relatively overlooked group of social fathers (O'Brien, 2011; Tarrant, 2013) whose involvement as primary caregivers can be essential in keeping children in family contexts. A raft of literatures, including those reviewed in Chapters 3 and 4, highlight that caregiving in later life can present specific challenges for older men (for example, Calasanti, 2004; Milligan and Morbey, 2016; Robinson et al, 2014). Not only are they marginalised by gender as male caregivers but they may also need to balance an increasing and unanticipated range of responsibilities. As O'Brien elaborates (2011: 111):

> as the later life course becomes more extended, varied and complex, men may begin to have overlapping multiple opportunities and obligations with respect to family and work. For example, grandfathering may coexist with employment, and the active parenting of a new set of children. Older men will face challenges in confronting earning and care responsibilities on multiple fronts, resulting in an expansion of the category 'double front' family. (Kröger and Sipila, 2005)

Other than some early research on older men, male kin and grandfathers by Sarah Cunningham-Burley (1984), overall, there has been a low critical mass of academic and policy research on their family participation and contributions. These omissions have been addressed during the 2010s to some extent, although the empirical basis for these findings is largely middle-class and resourced families (for example, Buchanan and Rotkirch, 2016; Mann et al, 2016; Tarrant, 2013; for an exception in the Finnish context see Timonen, 2020).

Recent sociological literatures examining the roles of grandparents reveal an important ethic of care that many grandparents demonstrate towards their grandchildren, including variation in the extent of childcare that they provide (Tarrant et al, 2017). Evidence suggests that this is no different for grandfathers who express the emotional significance of being a grandparent (Mann et al, 2016). Care provision for grandchildren is also variously shaped by different welfare state contexts (Herlofson and Hagestad, 2012), diverges across societal contexts and ranges within individual family contexts from legal guardianship to occasional caring (Mitchell, 2007). Demographic changes linked to ageing populations are also placing additional pressures on grandparent generations who may also be part of a sandwich generation and caring for their own parents as well as working and caring for grandchildren (Wellard, 2012; Ben-Galim and Silim, 2013).

The concept of ambivalence has been employed to explain the tensions and contradictions that exist in grandparents' explanations of normative expectations associated with their role as grandparent (that is, grandparenthood) and the realities of their roles (that is, grandparenting as social practice) (Tarrant et al, 2017). There are important class-based distinctions here too. Where middle-class grandparents report 'leisure/pleasure' grandparenting (Mason et al, 2007), characterised by 'being there' for children but 'not-interfering' with the expectations of parents, in low-income localities grandparents engage in 'rescue and repair' grandparenting (Hughes and Emmel, 2011; Emmel, 2017). Vulnerable and marginalised themselves, these grandparents provide supplementary and time-intensive care that is often invisible beyond the family and often results in complex and difficult engagements and dependencies on health and social care providers. As kinship carers with varying legal status determining the extent of parental responsibility they have for grandchildren (or other family members), these grandparents provide essential support on behalf of the state and often do so in contexts of significant economic hardship (see also Hunt, 2018).

In academic and policy research, the experiences of kinship carers are largely understood from the perspectives of women. However, MPLC accessed a hidden population of men providing essential care to children to sustain their families. Six of the MPLC participants were kinship carers and had various levels of social services involvement. Four were grandfathers (three maternal, one paternal) aged between 51 and 57, one was an uncle (maternal side), age 38, and one was a great-grandfather (maternal side), age 73. Of these, three had secured a care order and three were in the process of doing so (Table 5.3).

Despite being more resourced in general than the young fathers in the study, these men still described precarious relations with the labour market and were all living on a low income because they had taken on unexpected care responsibilities for younger family members in their mid-to late life. Those who were better resourced had a more secure home, were in relationships and had secure, legal care arrangements. Providing

Table 5.3: Kinship carer status and family configurations

Name	Age	Generational position	Kinship care status	Relationship status
Dougie	73	Great-grandfather	Special Guardian for two grandchildren	Married (second wife)
Paul	52	Grandfather	Special Guardian for three grandchildren	Lone father
Pearce	57	Grandfather	Special Guardian for three grandchildren	Married (primary carer)
Reggie	55	Grandfather	Special Guardian for two grandchildren	Married (secondary carer)
Sam	51	Grandfather	Seeking Special Guardianship Order for one grandson (Wave 1, secured by Wave 2)	In a relationship but lone father
Theo	38	Uncle	Informal carer seeking Special Guardianship Order for two of four nieces and nephews	Married (living apart while negotiating formal care status)

care to multiple, often traumatised and grieving children required a huge amount of emotional investment, skill and perseverance that the men who participated in MPLC appeared capable of providing. The narratives of two grandfathers, Sam and Paul, aged 51 and 52 and both lone (grand) fathers, respectively, are analysed here as exemplars of the lengths to which some men go to support and provide for their children and grandchildren.

Sam, a lone father and kinship carer to his grandson Leo, was accessed via the kinship care support team. His narrative predominantly focuses on his journey to securing responsibility for his very vulnerable grandson (aged four at the time of the interview) via a Special Guardianship Order. His son, the father of his grandson, still resides with him because he has learning difficulties and continues to require significant support as a young adult. Sam spent a great deal of time discussing the family trajectory of his grandson and the process of fighting to secure a safe upbringing for him with his paternal family.

The extent of the grandson's vulnerability was such that he was released into the care of his mother and maternal grandmother as a premature baby, weighing under 2lbs at birth. Sam described the mother of his grandson as 'streetwise', drawing on the 'shirker/scrounger' discourse so successfully weaponised within narratives of austerity to harden public attitudes towards welfare and benefits claimants (Patrick, 2015; Shildrick, 2018), especially lone mothers. Sam claimed that she had used his son to secure housing and welfare support. Later in the interview he revealed that both she and her eight siblings were also care experienced. Grandson

Leo presents with signs of abuse not long after his release to the home of his mother and maternal grandmother. He was returned to hospital with green-stick fractures and signs of neglect. Sam, who had been raising concerns daily with social services about his grandson, described a complicated and drawn-out process in which he attempted to report this abuse and secure primary care responsibility for Leo.

Sam experienced significant barriers in encouraging social services to consider him as a potential and competent carer for his grandson. He claims that in one exchange with a social worker it was suggested that they could not be sure that Sam himself had not been the person to cause the abuse, constructing him as potential risk. Much like the surveillance practices often observed by young fathers in contexts where social services intervene (Neale and Davies, 2015b), Sam was subject to suspicion at a crucial time in which Leo was being abused in the context of his maternal family.

In hindsight, Sam considered this to be an understandable caution, but his journey to securing legal guardian status was difficult. As his background in supporting his local community by taxiing young people and mentoring young people though boxing became clearer, he eventually got backing from the courts. He said of social services: "they didn't know I had all this background, you see. So when it went into court, or by the time it got to court, they were actually backing me." He described feeling shut out by social services and increasingly pushed towards the justice system.

These experiences of exclusion were compounded further by gendered thinking expressed by social workers. While Sam was the most resourced and capable individual in the wider family to care for his vulnerable grandson, he explained that during one assessment a social worker had visited his home and raised concerns about his ability to provide a good home. Her comments reflect the gendered thinking that pervades professional support, described in Chapter 4.

> ' "Right ok, something else that might go against you ..."
> she starts throwing all these things up. She said it was a very manly house. I said that there was flowers in the vase. She said it was full of boys. And I said, "Of course, I ain't got no daughters.' I asked if she wanted me to put make-up on and do me hair, and to tell me what she meant by that. She just said it didn't matter.' (See also Figure 5.1)

By the time of a second, follow-up interview, Sam had gained a Special Guardianship Order and he described how, despite the financial

Figure 5.1: A very manly house

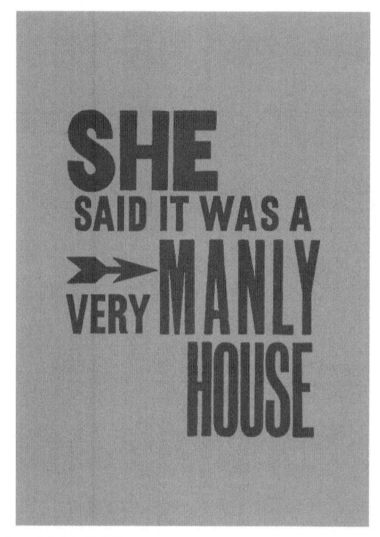

Source: © Katie Smith 2017

constraints created by taking on this extra responsibility, providing a secure home for his grandson had been emancipatory and his life had been transformed. To interpret his own circumstances, he compared himself to other men of his generation:

> '[Grandson] has changed my life entirely. Now it has made me more successful in every department … I think with him [grandson], yeah it's hard work, but – it sounds funny,

this – it stops you ageing. It definitely has ... definitely stopped me ageing ... I mean, I've got pals now that have been working their way over to the local working men's club, that's not living, is it? You know what I mean? [Laughter]'

Like lone father Rory, Paul, age 52, also described the high level of skill required to support children with complex needs, especially when those children have grown up in contexts of deprivation and have known other adverse childhood experiences.[4] Paul became a kinship carer to three of his grandchildren (two girls and a boy), following the death of his daughter with cancer when she was just 32. Paul's ex-partner was also incapable of providing for these children because of her own disability, and died not long after her daughter. Social services approached Paul, as their only remaining relative, to take on their care. However, because he was living in a two-bedroomed council house at the time only his two granddaughters could move in with him. This was linked to the same legalities described by Shane about how looked after children should be safely housed; namely, sisters are not allowed to share a bedroom with brothers. Despite the trauma of losing his mother, Paul's grandson was separated from his sisters and placed in a children's home, as had also been experienced by the young man Ashley, considered earlier in this chapter. Paul described a protracted process to request a larger home via the local authority so that he could look after all three children together, but was told that there was not enough available housing. At the time of the interview his grandson was in prison, having become involved in a cycle of criminality. Paul attributed this to 'the system', which he deemed to have failed both his grandchildren and himself. It is worth reiterating here that his grandson's trajectory, while described from Paul's perspective, is remarkably similar to that of Ashley.

The interview took place at Paul's new, larger council house which has enough rooms for all three of his grandchildren, including his grandson when he is out of prison. Much like Rory, Paul likens his care responsibilities for his very troubled and traumatised grandson to a poorly paid form of employment that nonetheless requires specific skills and experience (see also Tarrant, 2018):

'It's so frustrating for people. I mean, this is my case. I don't know about other people ... I mean, for me, to look after [grandson] in a professional capacity, I'd have to go to college to look after him, every week for four years to look after him, and I can still do it. They expect me to do it with no qualifications. It's like asking me to go and do a doctor's job, isn't it?'

Developing a gendered analysis, Milligan and Morbey (2016) suggest that unpaid caring can present men with a challenge to their masculinity, which they address by employing a strategy whereby they professionalise and thus legitimise their caring role. With reference to the skills and level of training required to support a young person with extensive and complex needs, Paul constructs care as work and emphasises the extent to which his role as a kinship carer is both financially and socially undervalued and afforded limited social status.

Paul's case further demonstrates the complex relational impacts of deprivation that have ripple effects across generations when young people, in this case a young man, are deprived of a secure home, separated from family and placed in the care system. While engagements with the criminal justice system are not inevitable for young, working-class boys, they are probable. The work of Maguire (2020), for example, indicates that for young men who grow up in contexts of deprivation there is evidence of similar gendered and classed trajectories that lead to 'revolving door' incarceration (Maguire, 2020). At a particularly challenging time when Paul was asked to keep his family together, he was rendered powerless by a complex set of legal requirements, expectations, poor funding and an increasingly punitive housing welfare system. These processes, observable within Paul's narrative and those of the other young men among the MPLC participants, also have specific longitudinal and intergenerational consequences that play out across families and impact on their resources.

Men who were married or living with partners also described how gendering processes linked to child protection legalities impacted on their relationships with their partners. As discussed in Chapter 4, male kinship carers may be especially vulnerable to accusations of sexual misconduct. State-imposed rules around the organisation of households that must be adhered to by family members in order to accommodate looked after children therefore have gendered implications. Both great-grandfather Dougie and grandfather Reggie and his wife Jane, for example, reflected on the impacts of state-imposed rules on them:

Reggie: We were told you can't do this or that.
Jane: We were told you can't leave them alone. If I went to the toilet I had to take the baby with me. That's how they made you feel. I didn't trust Reggie with the boys

at one point. That's how they made you feel ... it's weird because you are a kinship carer before you are a grandparent. That is how you are. I found that hard. They are my grandkids, you can't tell me what to do with them. Reggie gets a bit fed up with it. Social services. He knows we can't do owt about it. But it don't stop him having a whinge. He's opened up more. He didn't used to say owt. He just went with the flow.

...

Dougie: You have to be more aware of potential allegations; with a little girl in particular. I have to knock on the door before I go into the bedroom. With your own kids, it wouldn't cross your mind.

Anna: Does this worry you?

Dougie: No. I suppose because I'm confident that it won't happen. It is just that thought in the back of your mind. As they get older; if you had a big row with them about something. That is when things like that can potentially happen. You still have that in the back of your mind all the time.

The risk framework described here is pervasive in child protection contexts (Ladlow and Neale, 2016), and in the context of kinship care it seeps into private familial spaces and needs to be personally managed by these men and their families.

While there was a lot of discussion of risk, upheaval and negotiation among the kinship carers, particularly where men were caring for multiple children, the participants did describe some benefits of gaining new responsibilities. Despite the stress that reduced employment opportunities and financing can cause, the positive involvement of men in care is known to have wider implications for the broader societal project of gender equality. Shared responsibilities for care can help to reduce gender stereotypes and encourage mutual respect in relationships between men and women. Despite his annoyance at the required state intervention, Pearce, age 57, and his wife are key examples in this regard. When child protection concerns were raised about two of their grandchildren, aged two and four, and they were contacted by social services, Pearce and his wife had to decide how they would manage the new responsibilities. Pearce had worked for many years as a lorry driver and his wife was working successfully as a pharmacist after a long period as primary caregiver to their children. Pearce decided to leave his job to take on the primary care responsibility for his grandchildren.

While Pearce and his wife do not share care equally, the work/care role reversal of Pearce and his wife has given him valuable insights into the daily stresses of raising young children. As he reflects here, this new awareness means that he and his wife have developed a more understanding relationship based on shared experience:

> 'I were having a stressful job. So I just said right, I will jack it in. I'll look after the kids, but it were a massive learning curve because I've never done it before. I mean, when my kids were growing up, I were working on nights for nine years and I went full time on days but I never had to deal with small ones. At the time, my kids were nine and ten when I came off nights. So it were a massive learning curve for me and really, really hard. I can see what women sort of complain about when they've got kids round their feet all day and it's nice when my wife comes home. We get these to bed and we can talk and I've got adult conversation.'

In Pearce's case, the decision to become a main carer was motivated by a pragmatic and practical decision linked to the employment fortunes of the couple. As a partner in one of the more resourced and financially stable couples, Pearce gained insights about the gendered and emotional labour inherent in the provision of care, resulting in a renewed respect for his wife and an understanding relationship. However, in a second interview the benefits of becoming a carer were increasingly under threat. Like Sam, as the financial entitlements attached to the Special Guardianship Order were coming to an end Pearce came under increasing pressure from social services to find employment and was struggling to secure flexible and well-paid work at the age of 57. This point is examined further in Chapter 6.

The insights from these interviews confirm that male kinship carers experience many of the same kinds of issues that are already reported in the academic literature about grandparental experiences of kinship care, albeit predominantly drawing on women's views. While these men (and in some cases with their partners) were providing relatively stable placements, kinship care is a poverty trigger. The financial support attached to legal orders is inadequate and time limited, meaning that male kinship carers are at risk of, or experience, economic hardship. They also take on their role at great personal risk because of gendered and sexualised assumptions and legalities that govern men's responsibilities in intimate and private contexts. In combination, these processes can work against progress towards gendered transformations within family contexts; progress that is evidently possible, as several of these participants' narratives exemplify.

Concluding remarks

In this chapter, the diverse caring arrangements that characterise men's family participation in low-income families and contexts have been explored, demonstrating how men are involved in families, at what points in the lifecourse and in which ways. Their experiences reflect the dynamic character of family configurations in low-income contexts over time and how these are integral to the diverse lifecourse transitions of men in low-income and vulnerable family contexts. The cases in this chapter demonstrate a clear disconnect between individualising public and policy representations of marginalised fathers and families living in poverty which construct them as absent, uncaring and responsible for the perpetual transmission of poverty and deprivation. Certainly, the diverse caring arrangements and caring masculinities described uncover a wide range of emotional and material investments and interventions that are made by men in these contexts to sustain families.

Given the orientation of the study, many of the older men in the sample were primary caregivers, some of whom were engaging in care for young people who were traumatised and struggling with their own trajectories through deprivation. Notably, similar situations were also in evidence among the young fathers too. The pressures of maintaining family life in these circumstances are apparent in the men's narratives and they notably drew on discourses of coping and 'getting on' to demonstrate their capabilities to provide care in constrained financial circumstances. However, while caring may be unanticipated for some, it can also provide opportunities for forging new relationships, connections and forms of family engagement. In some instances, men also actively sought to secure care responsibilities via court processes in ways that speak in direct contradiction to policy discourses about feckless or absent men.

The complexity of these family forms and different and intersecting experiences of social marginalisation (like being deemed too young, too manly, too old; being a lone parent; or experiencing any combination of poor or inadequate housing; experiencing disability; and/or poor physical and/or mental health), also created conditions that impinged both on men's opportunities to provide care and their relationships in various ways. The experiences of the young fathers illustrate these findings especially. These young men were often the most marginalised and multiply disadvantaged in terms of their age, limited opportunities for secure employment, chaotic family backgrounds and poor housing, and had accrued the least resources over time. In combination, these circumstances meant that, compared to men in different age cohorts, they had the least opportunities available to them to engage in caregiving and take up responsibilities for their children. Yet, family participation for these young men also often took the form of engaging in intragenerational exchanges of care and support for younger siblings or wider family members like nephews and nieces. Thus, despite a multitude of factors mitigating against their efforts for their families, the participants demonstrated a strong commitment to those whom they were or felt responsible for. Nevertheless, the risk framing of men that is so pervasive in child protection contexts and that is applied regardless of their generational position or socioeconomic resources is also a key contextual constraint that was experienced across the MPLC sample.

Evidence in this chapter therefore demonstrates that orientations towards caregiving by men in these families were apparent but shaped predominantly out of changes in the material circumstances of families both within and across generations, either through a divorce or separation or through the death or incapacity of family members or partners with dependent children. Caring opportunities for these men arose out of these changes and prompted responses by them to attend to the needs of younger family members. This was despite the personal risks this might engender, such as becoming impoverished, being considered a risk by statutory agencies or being tipped into circumstances of marginalisation. Based on this evidence, family processes and trajectories should be considered more of an accumulation of events, changes and continuities over time rather than sudden 'turning' or 'trigger points'. I suggest that these processes also offer a more comprehensive explanation of how and why men participate in low-income families while also widening the empirical lens to a wider set of fathering in diverse social situations.

6

Familial economic circumstances and provisioning practices

'£3.26 to clothe five kids.'

When Theo, age 39, made this point in his interview for the MLPC study, he was providing informal kinship care to his niece, great-niece (aged 16 and 1) and nephews (aged 19, 8 and 5) following the death of his sister at the age of 32, and of his father 16 months prior to that. He had left employment to provide care for his two youngest nephews, one of whom has suspected learning difficulties, and was living for five days a week in his sister's rented accommodation. The five children mentioned here did not include his son, aged 12, and stepson, aged 2, whom he saw only at irregular weekends when he was able. While a decision was being determined by social services about whether he would obtain a care order for his two youngest nephews, he was paying for this house out of his now depleted life savings and with some money borrowed from his mother. His mother, aged 61, has Crohn's disease and was incapable of providing care for the children. When he did spend weekends with his partner, son and stepson he had to rely on his eldest nephew and niece to look after the two youngest children. He explained that he felt like he was being forced by social services into securing a Special Guardianship Order because, in his view and in the longer term, this was cheaper for the local authority. While all this was happening (over the school summer holidays) he had just £3.26 a day to support all five children, not including his own.

Theo's quote has been used to open this chapter because it so effectively illustrates the key themes explored both in the research and this book. It demonstrates, albeit in one of the more extreme of situations, how both financial and emotional pressures infuse the process of decision making around appropriate and necessary caring arrangements to keep children in families. Theo's family participation was contingent on his being the most resourced and capable person in his family to support these children and because he was regarded as the best-placed family member to ensure that the two younger children

Figure 6.1: £3.26 to clothe 5 kids

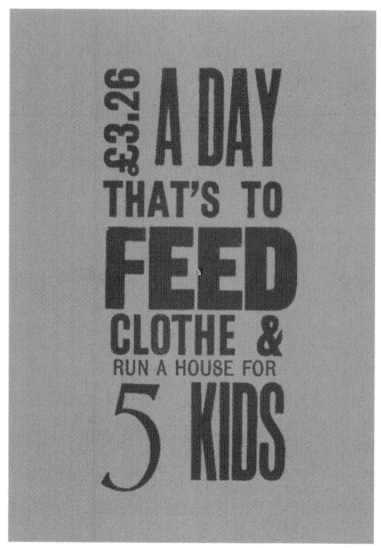

Source: © Katie Smith 2017

remained in the family. Yet, to do so came at an immense financial and personal cost for him. He had been forced out of employment to provide this care and was not in receipt of any state support while social services negotiated a new arrangement. Despite trying to keep these grieving children together and in the family, while also grieving himself, he was also plunged into poverty and forced to split his time and resources between two households. Both financial and emotional state support were severely lacking and inadequate for addressing the complexities of this family's structure and circumstances.

Taking Theo's account as a starting point, this chapter explores the financial constraints and barriers that impinge on men's efforts to participate in and preserve their families. Particular attention is paid to the ways in which money troubles and concerns about everyday finances influenced men's practices and decision making. Two main concepts are applied to explain these findings. First, building on feminist economist interventions, the concept of provisioning (Neysmith et al, 2010; Doucet, 2020) is employed to theorise the range of recognised and invisible relational strategies and practices that these men engage in so as to meet their responsibilities, secure an adequate income for their family and ensure safety for their children. According to Neysmith et al (2010), visible strategies of provisioning include engaging in formal and informal work in the labour market; providing caring labour in the domestic sphere; and undertaking community-based commitments. Less visible provisioning might include sustaining health; making claims external to families to assert rights; and ensuring safety. These provisioning practices reflect the variety of ways that men in low-income families 'do kinship'. Where Neysmith et al (2010) develop the concept to describe the kinds of gendered work that women predominantly do in the contemporary moment, this concept has sufficient depth to capture the broad range of activities that the men in this study described doing on behalf of their families both because they were doing so in the context of a low-income and because of necessity based on the nature of their responsibilities and family configurations.

I also place these insights in conversation with a burgeoning interdisciplinary scholarship that establishes how the familial and the financial are interconnected (Daly and Kelly, 2015; Hall, 2016a, 2016b, 2019), to examine men's family participation as infused with financial concerns constitutive of the conditions of low-income. Particular attention is paid to how they manage on their current income, and the extent of their exposure and vulnerabilities to financial shocks resulting from instabilities produced through caregiving, risk of debt and money worries.

The chapter is structured around the temporal perspectives of the participants, focusing first on the everyday challenges of trying to reconcile either insecure, low paid and inflexible work or the social security system with their care responsibilities. Consideration is also given to men's interactions with welfare processes, which have become increasingly punitive under the austerity-driven welfare regime that characterises the contemporary policy context. These findings are illustrative of the kinds of earning and caring trajectories that are affected by the increasing precarity of the local labour market and the conditionality of the welfare system, which can sometimes trigger crisis and unexpectedly push families into poverty (for example, Hughes and Emmel, 2011). Finally, attention is given to how men anticipate and imagine their personal welfare futures and those of their families under austerity.

Reconciling earning and caring

The ability to provide financially for children is a pressing concern for all fathers, but is more so for low-income fathers. As noted in Chapter 3, practices of 'caring' and 'earning' are intertwined and are central aspects of fathering identities. Being a financial provider is also intimately bound up with ideals of good fatherhood and male identity (Neale and Davies, 2015a). The reconciliation of employment and care responsibilities was therefore a juggle for the participants interviewed for MPLC, but especially for those who had primary care responsibilities. Other than the older men in the sample, few had any experience in their lifecourse of secure long-term employment, meaning that financial provisioning was inaccessible and problematic. Instead, they described complex longer-term work trajectories demarcated by tenuous access to the labour market. This has variable longitudinal and generational effects.

Evidence suggests that recessionary processes have disproportionately impacted on young people in the domain of employment. Young people describe difficulties in entering and navigating the labour market, and when they are in jobs they are more likely to lose them (Hogarth et al, 2009). The education, training and employment pathways of young fathers are also variable and shaped by a constellation of life circumstances (Neale and Davies, 2015a). These challenging work trajectories and employment conditions were reflected in the narrative of Ashley, the young man living with his sister and nephew (see Chapter 5). Here he describes the juggle of balancing insecure work with family. Two weeks prior to the first interview, Ashley had started a job doing fundraising for a national charity. He was paid £7 per hour for his work, and he described it as "hard-core". He explained that he did more than five hours of work a day but got paid for only the five. He was critical of the work, which involved asking for money on people's doorsteps late at night:

> 'I'm knocking on people's doors asking for them to donate
> at nine o'clock at night. I said it might seem all right to you

lot, but I said it's not right. I said between eight o'clock and nine o'clock, everyone's just whinging about what time it is. I said between eight o'clock and nine o'clock every door that I knock on just say "no, have you seen the time?" And I'm like yeah, sorry, but I have to. I have to ... I miss putting him to bed and that as well [pointing to Caid].'

Like many of the participants in the study, Ashley was keenly aware of public and political representations of low-income families as shirkers, characterising the political register of austerity. Where policy would have it that worklessness is the product of individual inefficiencies, Ashley, who was working in highly insecure and commission-based employment, highlighted the distinct lack of support available to achieve his aspirations for a family, secure home and employment. Referring to the government position on employment he said:

'They keep saying that you need to do this, you need to do that. We all want to do that. They're acting like we don't want to do it when we do. I want to work. I want a decent house. I want kids, everything, you know what I mean? But it's having help doing that.'

With remarkable similarities, young father Joe was also eloquent about the complexities involved in sustaining insecure and exploitative employment over time, especially as a new parent:

'When I was 21, I had three jobs in a year and a half. This was after my little boy. I had my own place and that. So I started working and that. My first job I ended up leaving because I thought I was rich. The second one I got pulled in about my criminal record. I was only there four days. I couldn't do nothing about that because I was doing door to door. Home fundraising. And basically I got caught on the same day I had to go to work. He [manager] pulled me into the office and spoke to me. I think I should have gone round it another way. I think if I'd gone around it another way and said something else but I just told him. What we'll do he said because I was doing door to door sales, for [major charity] ... before he told me he had to sack me, he said get all this out the way and go to court and jail if you have to and at the end come back and I'll give you a job. After I got everything out the way I ended up getting myself back into trouble again.'

The narratives of Ashley and Joe demonstrate a clear example of what MacDonald and Shildrick (2018) term 'conventional aspirations' towards the package deal of employment, family and house (Townsend, 2002). Bearing remarkable similarity to the narratives of other disadvantaged young men who have participated in studies examining social exclusion and policy (MacDonald and Shildrick, 2018), such aspirations are 'stubbornly normal' aspects of young people's transitions to adulthood, and persist despite the realities of the contemporary labour market. Evidence presented in Chapter 3 suggests that young fathers in a range of international and socially disadvantaged contexts express a distinct desire to be involved in their children's lives while also fulfilling the prerogative of providing for them economically (Neale and Davies, 2015a). However, the 'low pay, no pay cycle' (Shildrick et al, 2012) they describe here mitigates against their efforts and impinges directly on their family lives and investments. Their commitment to a normative lifecourse endures nonetheless, even when exploitative and insecure work and unemployment impacts on their abilities to adhere to the broader cultural ethos of engaged fatherhood (Neale and Patrick, 2016).

Joe's narrative further indicates that such issues are also magnified for disadvantaged young men with experience of the criminal justice system (Ladlow and Neale, 2016). Despite being offered some support by his employer, the complex mix of Joe's chaotic family background, history of being both victim and perpetrator of domestic violence, and of reoffending, made it difficult for him to prioritise and hold down employment, impacting on his ability to fulfil his intentions to be there for his youngest child.

Reflecting generational differences in the impact of socioeconomic restructuring, older men have been described as more likely to be disadvantaged by a lack of flexibility in terms of contracted hours (Yeandle et al, 2003). While unemployment is often considered to be a problem for young men, in the year 2000 in the UK, one third of British men not in employment were aged between 50 and 65, meaning that some 2.5 million were economically inactive and reliant on state or private benefits in some form (McDowell, 2000). Recent data suggests that male economic inactivity rates for this age group have remained largely constant since 1984 (Department for Work and Pensions, 2018).

The employment biography of Matthew reflected this wider national employment picture and the effects on the locality where he lived, which was characterised by the decline of manufacturing work and widespread deindustrialisation (Nayak, 2006) that has affected many northern English cities. Having lost his job at a local and well-known clothes-manufacturing factory which closed, Matthew experienced a much longer-term pattern of unemployment compounded by his role as a carer for his adult disabled son. He was recruited to MPLC via a major charity in the city, who suggested that he regularly 'pestered' them for flexible work opportunities that would accommodate the needs of his son. Here he describes his frustrations in trying to secure employment:

'This is why it's frustrating. Even this [charity] job. It's either 21 hours or 28 hours. This morning I've just dropped him [disabled son] off at this centre. He officially doesn't start till 10 am. From 9:30 am to get to [nearby city], you'd be struggling for 10 am. Then I have to pick him up at 3:30 pm. They'd say "well you can get transport". The transport is so erratic. It was either not turning up or turning up at 10:30am. So I said to them what are you going to say if you get a job "Oh I'm sorry I can't get in today till 12pm." You've no option but taking yourself. There's never been any funding for Friday. So any job would have to be Monday to Thursday. And you are looking at that time-scale of hours. It's frustrating. The government makes out that everyone wants to be out of work. Stay on welfare benefits. They make it so difficult.'

Time is a finite resource for many families, but the negotiation of Matthew's individual and intersecting routines with those of his son was a real issue. Matthew's troubles in securing flexible work are also mirrored by fathers already in employment. According to research by Olchawski (2016) and Working Families (2017), fathers are more likely than mothers to have their requests for flexible work refused and fear that such requests are likely to be more damaging to their careers. While the employment trajectories of Ashley and Joe reflect young fathers' struggles with low-paid, exploitative work, so too do those of older lone fathers. Combined with the narratives of Ashley and Joe there is ample evidence to suggest here that, regardless of generational position, men feel let down by increasingly punitive government policy and expectations and organisational cultures that are inflexible and/or exploitative. These mitigate against their efforts both towards securing and sustaining employment and their family responsibilities.

Not only this, but the participants also had to make otherwise relatively invisible claims on a regular basis to a variety of support services or government agencies. This included any combination of welfare and social assistance services, public housing, the court system, the education and health sectors, child protection agencies and other community-based services. Like the families interviewed for the IGE legacy study, the MPLC data was saturated with accounts of profound uncertainties, vulnerabilities and risks associated both with accessing health and social care services and with professional service involvement. This was especially the case for the kinship carers once they had acquired parental responsibility for their grandchildren. According to Emmel and Hughes (2014), kinship care represents an intensification of reliance on formal and voluntary service provisions. Those men who had primary parental responsibility for their children were therefore very active in engaging with services to broker resources. However, as noted in Chapter 4, getting help or support was rarely uncomplicated (Emmel and Hughes, 2014), and many of the kinship carers felt sidelined and short-changed by social services. Reggie, for example, describes a lack of transparency about what he and his wife are entitled too: "It's been five years and we have just found out we could have a car off them. And no one told us in five years. We just found out by someone [another kinship carer] who gets one every year." Pearce and Sam also described concerns about the expectations placed on carers to balance meaningful employment with their care responsibilities, and the need to access resources and support in order to demonstrate the legitimacy of their claims about living in hardship as produced by their new familial arrangements. Pearce explained:

'We struggle. This is why I am going back to see [social services] in September. We get this income support but because I can't claim anything, but they will ask me to get a job; and I can't because I have two kids to look after. Have to get this family credit thing: £300 a month. I know I've got a job if I want it. I'm going to try and get a job at a friend's company: delivering beds. I'm hoping that he will let me have all the holidays off or it is no good to me. I cannot afford to put these in [childcare] full time ... if they are off for six weeks in holiday, it will cost me more than I can earn. This will be £70 a day. Childcare is £10 per afternoon each. £7.50 per morning: a couple of hundred pound a week; and I am going to earn £100. If they will let me come and work for him five days a week and have weekends off and holidays. If that works, brilliant. If it don't, I don't know what I will do.'

Sam also described the uneasy relationship that kinship carers with Special Guardianship Orders have with the state and the competing expectations that they should fulfil their citizenship not only as caregivers but also as workers (see Chapter 5). In a follow-up phone call with him he explained that he had been granted a Special Guardianship Order in November 2016. However, this had pushed him into debt, posing further constraint on his income. At the time of gaining the order, social services had asked him to give up work to settle his grandson so as to give him time to adjust. Once secured, they then asked Sam how he was going to continue to afford providing care for his grandson without employment. Effectively, once the Special Guardianship Order was granted Sam became a job seeker again and his move to Special Guardianship Order recast his status as a kinship carer with protected status back to a worker again. Where he had been claiming Family Tax Credits, he was then informed he must now claim Working Tax Credit. He was also told by the council that he was over-claiming for his other son who was living with him. They informed him that he owed them £7,000 in overpaid money. This lack of clarity on the part of the council meant that Sam was in a serious amount of debt without being aware. The complexities of his status led him to ask, "Am I a worker, a job seeker, or a government employee?" Despite Sam's engaging in vital care and support on behalf of the state to keep his grandson in the family, his account demonstrates that the citizenship of individuals who become state ratified as kinship carers is uneasy and opaque.

Suggesting that this might be a wider issue, grandfather Andrew, age 70, who was accessed via the community centre, also demonstrated an uncomfortable transition back to employment, having spent many years as a carer, first for his father-in-law and then as a primary caregiver for his step-children. Andrew also has a heart problem, which places limitations on opportunities for meaningful employment. Discussing his failed attempts to re-enter the labour market and experiences of stigmatisation by employers, he explained: "this is how your career goes down because you can't get – nobody wants you. 'Are you employed?' 'I'm a carer.' 'You must be a waste of space.'"

Managing 'shocks', and strategies for getting by

As noted in Chapter 4, Emmel and Hughes (2014) describe how families in low-income contexts can be easily tipped into crisis or shocks, especially when lacking access to adequate resource or support. Managing these shocks and navigating complex systems was a way in which men in low-income families described the 'doing' of family and kinship in ways that are less often disclosed by more resourced families. Several of the MPLC participants confirmed this finding, describing how they developed strategies for managing unanticipated bills or errors with welfare payments. Often this resulted in them having to go without themselves, and required extensive management strategies to address errors or to work with organisations.

This was described by Shaun, a lone father and primary caregiver to his two young daughters. He was particularly eloquent about the constraints of providing care under limiting financial circumstances. He was also one of the few men to agree to participate in the photovoice task (see Chapter 1). Involved in the pilot phase of the photovoice, Shaun used a disposable camera, which unfortunately affected the integrity of the data (Figure 6.2). Despite the poor quality of the image, in a follow-up interview he explained the gravity of what was depicted. An electricity and gas bill requesting payment of £735 that arrived just before Christmas:

'This was huge. This was a gas bill. And what's happened is, and they've done it again to me. Now what happened in December. They sent me a peculiar bill. Similar to this one. This is the latest one. Same thing as last time. Cancelled

Figure 6.2: An unexpected electricity bill; taken by Shaun

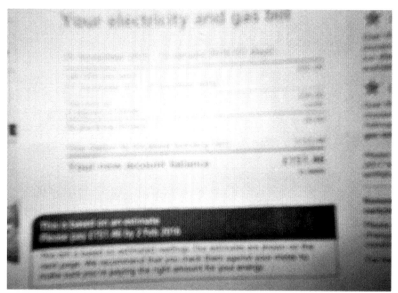

Source: © Anna Tarrant 2016

some charges for you. The last time it happened, I just paid it and crossed it off. And then a couple of weeks later the actual bill came. So I called them and said for my own part I apologise but I can't just come up with this money. They also, which is a good thing, periodically check whether there is a better price for me. Every couple of weeks. So I was about due for one of those letters. I thought that was what it was and I'd read it later. It turns out that this was just a statement. And the one on top of the fridge was a bill. So then no bill comes. And then I get a warning. So I immediately remember that letter and sure enough it was a bill for the £212. There's no way I could pay it or offer them anything. So they said "can you pay £7 every fortnight?" And I thought I could just about manage. The other idea was to come round and put a payment meter in and I said no. Because I know what that is. To put me on a more expensive tariff. And it alleviates you of your legal responsibility to provide my children with gas and electricity. Because in court they will say he cut himself off because he didn't top his meter up.'

When families experience financial pressures, they are often faced with determining how to put their children first (Ridge, 2009). This manifests in rational behaviour, including careful and painstaking planning about expenditure and prioritisations of need (Daly and Kelly, 2015; Hall, 2016a). Leisure and recreation activities are the first things to be cut, followed by essentials like heating, equipment, clothing and food. Unanticipated gas and electricity bills can also be further compounded by additional complications that result in debt in the worst cases. Such considerations may occasionally involve prioritising 'luxury' spending, preserving the socio-emotional, rather than the physical essence of family at certain times. In his follow-up interview, for example, Shaun further elaborated the need to rely on the financial support of his new girlfriend, Tara, when his housing benefits were stopped without his knowledge, so that he could provide for his daughters at Christmas:

Shaun: This was really bad. If it hadn't been for Tara, my girlfriend, Christmas probably wouldn't have happened. Just before Christmas the housing benefit decided to stop my benefit. They didn't tell the housing association as usual. First I heard about it was about four weeks before Christmas.

Housing association sent me a letter saying I was in serious rent arrears.

Anna: You told me about this because you were waiting to see if the payment was going to go in?

Shaun: And it never did and went on all the way through Christmas. I ended up in serious debt with the housing association and still am. I've got to pay a top-up because of the spare bedroom. I take that on the nose because I don't want to move the kids again after everything they have been through. That's what I have to do. The housing benefit situation carried through all the way through Christmas into January. It was mid-January when they sorted it out. At one point the housing association had to issue me with preliminary order for eviction.

Shildrick et al (2012) note that existing or new debts are rarely factored into welfare entitlements, which is problematic, especially when this places severe limitations on people's ability to purchase essential items including food, clothing and heating, and affects their everyday provisioning. These material and financial strains put additional pressures on parenting, due to the continual effort to make ends meet and budget (Ridge, 2009). Research with low-income families also suggests that parents report feeling under strain to buy expensive branded clothes and trainers for their children, fuelled by anxieties that their children will be bullied or marginalised if they do not wear the 'right' clothes (Ridge, 2009). In describing the needs of his granddaughter, kinship carer Paul made this same point, highlighting the hidden expenses implicated in bringing up a teenager:

'Well, I mean financially, you know, to look after a child. This is my view. I mean, I think I get tax credits for [granddaughter, age 13]. She isn't my child, if you understand what I mean? This is what I'm saying. If she was plonked in somebody else's house … they get fortunes for them, you know, and I think I get about 30 quid a week or something like that, to bring a 13-year-old child up. It costs me £95 for her trainers! [laughs]'

In identifying the cost of his granddaughter's shoes, Paul also compares his meagre financial entitlements to those of other legal care positions, like fostering. In families like Paul's, which have been formed out of necessity (in this case to keep his grieving grandchildren in the family), these financial limitations can make it particularly difficult to provision for, and manage the social and emotional lives of their children, who are already stigmatised for being raised by family members rather than parents.

It was also sometimes necessary for the participants themselves to go without. Sometimes this included luxuries, but occasionally it also meant doing without food. A common strategy discussed was to shop savvy, including buying food from the reduced-to-clear section of the supermarket (Figure 6.3). These are important financial management strategies often used by low-income families to negotiate hardships (McKendrick et al, 2003; Ridge, 2009). Matthew, for example took the photograph in Figure 6.3 on his shopping trip to demonstrate the everyday reality of hardship.

Andy and Dean, two dads I met at the community centre who were visiting to pick up some decorating items, also suggested that making their welfare payments last long enough (which they notably referred to as 'getting paid') is an active and temporally demarcated process that sometimes requires reliance on wider family members for financial support.

Figure 6.3: The 'reduced to clear' section of the supermarket; taken by Matthew

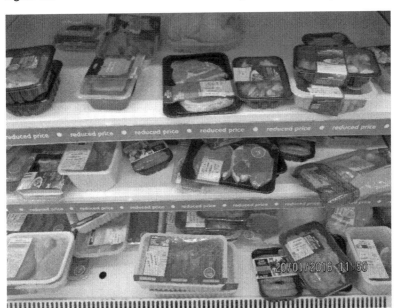

Source: © Anna Tarrant 2016

Andy: Usually with your money, you get your food and everything in right away, before you spend anything on yourself, because everything …

Dean: Whatever's left, is left.

Andy: [overlapping] Whatever's left, and it's not a great deal, it i'nt, you're lucky if he gets 15 quid or something income.

Dean: By the time we've done us shopping and paid electric and TV licence, cable bill, whatever else, there's not much left, but I always make sure when we go shopping we have enough to last us 'til next time we get paid. Always works out, 'part from Sunday can sometimes be a bad day but someone'll help me out, but my mum will help me out or our lass's mum will help me out.

Dean made it clear later in the interview, however, that financial dependencies and exchanges with wider family members were not preferable and could not be negotiated on a regular basis. They represented a form of exchange that they could not always reciprocate, resulting in relational tensions and social fragmentation, recognised in existing research with low-income families (Offer, 2012). This was a fear expressed by several of the participants.

Welfare trajectories and processes

As the comments by Andy and Dean indicate, for those men who were unemployed, family provisioning was reliant on increasingly punitive welfare payments and activities associated with searching for employment. Welfare support under austerity has become increasingly conditional on finding employment (Welfare Conditionality Project, 2018), regardless of care responsibilities or the ability to access affordable local childcare. Changes to the welfare system were having notable impacts on the men who were primary caregivers, all of whom were of working age. For the older of these men, such changes were intensified. Joseph, the 45-year-old father discussed in Chapter 5 had been workless for several years as a result. Changes to the welfare support system had proven to be challenging for him as a single father, and more so since the age of his eldest daughter meant that she no longer qualified for child benefit. He explained that since she turned 16 he had stopped receiving tax credits for her. Given the challenges young people now face in finding secure work, she did not earn her own wage and was dependent on her father for housing and financial support. Despite the many physical and emotional issues that he experienced because of his physical disability, Joseph explained that in a recent work capability test he had been deemed fit for work, causing him to lose his Employment and Support Allowance. The local housing association through which he was accessed for the study was supporting him to challenge the decision because there was very little work that he could physically do linked to his illness. He explained:

> 'All they [the job centre] said is, "Well you've got to look for work and you've got to apply for so many jobs", and I had got one person telling me I'd got to work from eight o'clock in the morning until half past three, and then one woman at the social when I was signing on said, "You need to work any of them."
>
> 'And I said, "Well what about my daughter coming home from school at three? She's 12 years old, she can't stay in the house on her own. If I leave her in the house on her own, I'm going to get arrested and get done and have her taken off me." And they said, "Well she'd be all right for half an hour or an hour."
>
> 'Apart from the problems that I've got looking for work is the hardest part of it. Like I say, if you don't look for work you get sanctioned and you lose half your benefits and when you've got kids you've got to … [unable to continue speaking].'

Joseph suggested that the 'social' would not make allowances for the fact that he was a single father who also needed to fit his time around his youngest daughter's school routine. His efforts to sustain a parental identity and responsibilities conflicted with requirements to become a worker. He was therefore caught in a structural tension between family and employment. His familial and biographical timescapes did not mesh with the requirements of other, statutory timescapes and practices (Emmel and Hughes, 2014; Tarrant and Hughes, 2020). Worryingly, he also described being actively encouraged by a statutory agency to leave his child alone so he would meet the requirements to find work that he was physically incapable of doing. Ironically, despite the pervasiveness of the risk framework in child protection contexts, as described in Chapter 5, he was asked to engage in risky family practices in order to fulfil his work placement requirements. The conflicting nature of these obligations therefore increased the vulnerability of this lone parent by obscuring and undermining his responsibilities to his child. This case is a clear example of how competing expectations produced by austerity-driven policy reform, especially in relation to employment and welfare, exacerbate the struggles of already vulnerable families, including one headed by a lone father who was living on a low income, was physically disabled and experiencing severe depression.

Child maintenance policy and processes

When fathers are non-resident, provisioning can involve financial transfers and exchanges across households. In many industrialised countries, child maintenance policy has been developed to secure the living standards of children following parental relationship dissolution. A key aspiration of child maintenance policy is to reduce the poverty experienced by children whose parents do not share a household (Hakovirta, 2011). This kind of financial provisioning has become increasingly necessary in the dual-earner household and policy context. Questions about child maintenance support were purposely built into the interview schedules for the study, driven by observations made unprompted by participants in IGE and FYF about financial obligations (Tarrant, 2017 and see Chapter 1). Such concerns were most relevant to the men who were non-resident or who had been through processes of divorce or separation, as opposed to the men who were resident, primary caregivers. So far, the interpretations developed in this chapter have illustrated the financial and practical challenges that these men faced in reconciling work and care and which underscored these financially precarious family contexts. As noted earlier, qualitative research indicates that there are gendered differences in how men and women respond to poverty, with men more likely to express feelings of shame, emasculation or gender role crisis (for example, Fodor, 2006; Bennett and Daly, 2014). In this study, however, these gendered aspects were not fully explicit in men's narratives. It was mainly in discussions around child maintenance that the active gendering of parenting and finances was perhaps most pertinent for these participants, especially in terms of perceived and actual inequities sustained through the redistribution of wealth and care responsibilities across households.

Of the men who expressed specific concerns about the child maintenance system, they confirmed its propensity to reinforce representations of absent, non-resident fathers in its emphasis on redistributing wealth to individuals claiming child benefits, usually mothers. For women, who are more likely to be lone parents, benefits paid for children can help to reduce mothers' poverty risk, and child maintenance payments are an important source of income to parents living below the poverty line. However, there is little evidence about the impact of the risk of poverty for non-resident parents (usually fathers) making these payments.

Rory, lone father and carer of his adult disabled son, raised specific concerns about the requirement to pay child maintenance in the early days following the breakdown of his marriage, despite providing three days of care a week for his son. He held primary parental responsibility for his son at the time of the interview but reflected retrospectively on his engagement with the then Child Support Agency, considering the way in which the agency positioned him. The Child Support Agency, which was reformed and renamed as the Child Maintenance Service in 2013, was originally established by the Conservative government in 1993, reflecting a new UK state interest in supporting families, albeit one that prioritised a focus on absent fathers and men's roles as financial providers rather than on female participation in the labour market (Eisenstadt and Oppenheim, 2019). As Gillies (2005) and Williams (2004) suggest, the Child Support Act 1989 aimed to make 'absent fathers' liable and accountable for the costs of their children, substituting welfare support with child maintenance as a private financial responsibility. This approach shifted financial liability away from the state to individuals and reinforced the centrality of breadwinning, rather than residence, as a vital aspect of the role of the biological father (see also Williams, 1998; Earley, 2017).

The most recent reforms to the system are premised on principles that encourage family-based arrangements whereby parents have the scope to make decisions about payments based on their own family circumstances, regardless of what the law prescribes (Bryson et al, 2015). Other than research by Bryson et al (2015), which explored how the British public perceived child maintenance and the current system and McHardy (2016), which examines issues of child maintenance for individuals and services within the Fife area in Scotland, there is limited research in the UK about the impacts of child maintenance requirements and arrangements on non-resident parents or those who have shared residency arrangements (e.g. Andreasson and Johansson, 2019). Demonstrating parallels with men's experiences of the Australian system (Natalier and Hewitt, 2010; 2014) and providing a rare account from the UK about post-separation arrangements and child maintenance support, MPLC revealed both the material and non-material reasons for men's dissatisfaction with this privatised system.

Rory was 61 and a single father and carer for his adult son, aged 30. He was of the view that the requirement to pay child support reinforced the absent father and father-as-financial-provider narrative at the expense of the wider, caring aspects of his role. This positioning is at odds with contemporary cultural imperatives associated with the involved father, as well as the expectations and constructions of fathering that men hold for themselves.

> 'I had to take her [son's mother] to court and get shared residence, and that cost me just short of £4,000 – well, just over £4,000. I had to get bank loans out for it and everything. It didn't cost her a bloody penny actually … You also have to pay maintenance and what have you. Even when I had shared residence – I had [disabled son] three days and she had him four – I had to give her maintenance for four days, but I couldn't claim maintenance for three days. Whoever holds the child benefit can claim maintenance. If you have the child one day a week and you got the child benefit, you could claim maintenance off the other person. It's wrong, and I argued that fact out with them, the Work and Pensions or whatever it is … they said it's how it works, it's better that way. And then [son] came to live with me when he was about 12. He kept saying to me, "Can I come and live with you?" and I said, "Well, of course you can. You can make the decision … and I thought, she's going to kick off, his mum, but yeah, fine.'

In the case of child maintenance, and in policy terms, there is a risk that fathers are explicitly addressed to make them financially accountable only when they are deemed to be 'absent' from households. This framing, which places emphasis on the biological connectedness of fathers and feeds a 'gender-divided idea of parenthood' (Andreasson and Johansson, 2019: 2), does not align with the diversity of contemporary families or the complex character of gendered relations between separated parents. Shaun, for example, made some especially astute comments about how child maintenance policies reinforce negative discourses and positions around separated parents. He proposed a hypothetical middle ground that would allow him and his ex-partner to come to their own financial arrangements in ways that were less punitive and would ensure that both parents were financially stable and that their children were best supported:

Shaun: There is no positive language around families who get on amicably. It all sounds like people are at each other's necks. Absolutely not what the norm is. Most families out there are like myself and [ex-partner]. We get on very well with each other ... the people who dole the benefits out, what they want to know is who the primary carer is. If I tell them I'm the primary carer but she's getting the benefits and giving half to me that then becomes fraudulent. I don't understand why that is. They wrote to me and asked me to tell them. Asking me to define percentages of time that the children are here with their mother and how many beds at their mother's. How many here? Who does the school run first if the child gets ill? I thought the questions were really peculiar. They made me feel weird about parenting my own children. They think of things I've never thought about.

Anna: Trying to quantify your relationship?

Shaun: Absolutely. Bring it down to numbers and figures. It's not possible.

Here, Shaun observed a dissonance between policy visions of normative family life and the messy, lived realities of familial and personal relationships as they are enacted across households. Shaun more generally held egalitarian views of his relationships with women and expressed this in terms of his priorities around support for his children (Figure 6.4).

Despite a shared dissatisfaction with how the child maintenance system operates and positions fathers as financially accountable and absent, Rory and Shaun approached the issue from different perspectives, informed by their differing familial, economic and interpersonal circumstances. Rory's relationship with his ex-partner was much more adversarial than Shaun's, for example, and he viewed the economic instability as an additional component of inequity in his relationship with his ex-partner. Nonetheless, both men prioritised the emotional ties and time spent with their children as vital and significant in ways that are obscured by policy interventions like this. For these men, the child maintenance system reinforced gendered inequalities and power dynamics between couples. These findings indicate a distinct lack of advice and information for separating families around child maintenance, as well as the complex and diverse ways families break down (McHardy, 2016).

While redressing these inequalities is clearly important, Featherstone (2009) cautions that the inequalities men experience within this context must be treated reflexively and in a way that rebalances inequalities that also impact on the lives of women. It is apparent that these 'fathers'

Figure 6.4: You've got to love your kids more than you dislike their mother

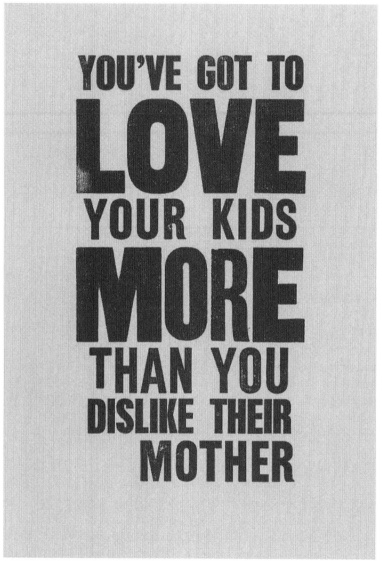

Source: © Katie Smith 2017

subjective aspirations and strivings are filtered through structural and cultural conditions in society' as Andreasson and Johansson (2019: 2) observe in the Swedish context. The MPLC findings suggest that current welfare policy in the UK continues to feed a gendered division of labour in parenting that does not align with those families where men share custody. While the men in MPLC were highly involved fathers, there is a risk that that when finances are prioritised over care, this may curtail the involvement of fathers altogether (Roy, 1999), with adverse effects for men, women and children.

Securing appropriate housing

Another key strategy employed by the men was securing appropriate housing, an emergent theme that was briefly considered in Chapter 5. Several of the participants were living in low-cost, run-down and inadequate housing in deprived neighbourhoods. The young fathers had the most insecure housing situations and most were experiencing or had experienced periods of homelessness. This was linked in part to how they were recruited, but also reflects broader findings (Neale and Ladlow, 2015). Three of the young dads were accessed via housing agencies and all three reported insecure tenancies and periods of housing insecurity. Those with the least secure housing trajectories were also the least connected to their children and saw them much less regularly.

The two young fathers who secured parental responsibility for their children via court processes, Shane and Ricky, described provisioning for their children in terms of securing appropriate social housing in the locality. Like the men's engagements with other support agencies, securing social housing was a lengthy process and there was little recognition of their roles as primary caregivers. As discussed in Chapter 5, once housing had been secured, things did not necessarily become any easier. In the case of Shane, for example, sanctions were inaccurately applied for the 'spare' bedroom in his home, linked to the introduction of the Bedroom Tax as part of the Welfare Reform Act 2012. Shane is the young father who was advised at the last minute about his paternity of his young son. Here he describes going without food when he moved into his council-owned home with his two children, but also indicates the pressure he was put under early in the process of moving into social housing to provide a suitable environment for his children.

> 'For the first week there was no boiler in because in new council houses now they take all the boilers out so they don't get pinched or damaged whilst there's nobody living there. So for the first week there wasn't a boiler but they charged me the first week's rent and they tried to charge me the Bedroom Tax for about two months, and again I had to go to the housing a few times to explain that

I wasn't paying that week's rent because there wasn't a
boiler in my house – there was no heating and no water
… anyway I ended up having to pay it because it was just
causing loads of problems so I thought I would just pay it.
I brought everything more or less brand new, I didn't have
any savings or anything to buy my things with so obviously
for the first couple of months I was lucky to live on one
meal a day, and I did lose quite a bit of weight doing it.'

Ricky, who had recently acquired primary responsibility for his young
daughter, experienced similar issues. When I visited his home for
interview there was minimal furniture, the walls were being painted
and he was acquiring carpets "on the cheap" via a known associate
in the locality. Despite the decoration being a work in progress, the
provisioning of a safe home and control over the environment he was
creating for his daughter was a significant source of pride for him.

In some instances, key workers and welfare officials subjected
the participants and their homes to social scrutiny and surveillance.
Surveillance in respect of property maintenance, domestic chores and
cleanliness has been identified as characteristic of the responsibilisation
agenda associated with the Troubled Families Programme (Bond-Taylor,
2016), a government-initiated programme in England that conducts
targeted interventions for families experiencing multiple disadvantages.
Darren, one of the young fathers interviewed for the FYF study in
2011, explained that the key role of his family support worker had been
"to monitor and make sure the house is perfectly clean and our son
perfectly tidy". Shaun described a similar visit from a housing officer,
explaining how she subjected his home to scrutiny and conflated her
perceptions of this environment with his abilities as a parent:

'I don't know how she became a housing officer. I don't
have a great deal nice to say about her. My mum always said
if you don't have something nice to say about somebody,
don't say it. She doesn't understand family life. She came
in once and said "You will have to clean all this off the
wall before you move out." I said you don't clean it, you
paint over it. I know where to get this paint, it's council
standard paint. It's not Dulux. Why is a housing officer
coming in and making comments about a one-year-old and
a two-year-old drawing on the wall? The reason I don't
have carpets is because I said I wouldn't till they are at least

eight or nine because I'll be doing it again. Because they just get spilt on.'

As noted in the previous chapter, appropriate housing was also essential to the grandparents and family members who became kinship carers. Lack of adequately sized housing resulted in splitting up a sibling group in Paul's case, and Sam's house was judged by a social worker as being 'too manly'. Kinship carer couple Reggie and Jane also described a difficult process that impinged heavily on their finances and required them to be rehoused outside of the area where they had grown up and established ties. They explained that when their grandsons Kyle and Kenan were dropped at their door with no clothes, they were given just £26 to purchase some nappies and milk for Kyle, the youngest. Their home, which had been adequate for the couple, could not accommodate the additional children. Indicating the size of their living room, where the interview took place and which could comfortably accommodate two three-seater sofas but little more, they explained:

Reggie: We were all in a room about half the size of this.
Jane: Two triple wardrobes. Two doors. Double bed.
            Bedside cabinets. And two cabin beds. We lived like
            that for eighteen months. And they moved us here.
            When we got the boys, we didn't get a link worker
            till the May. Got the boys in December. We didn't
            become kinship carers till September.

In reflecting on their house move, enforced by social services to provide more adequate space for them and their grandchildren, they said:

Jane: We had no choice about moving here. No choice.
Reggie: They weren't willing to help us with an extension.
Jane: They weren't even willing to find us a three-bedroom
            house over there. They just said 'Right that's where
            you are going.'
Reggie: I wouldn't take the garden away from them.
Jane: Don't get me wrong, its quiet but we have no family
            or friends here. They all live at that side.

This move isolated Reggie and Jane from their existing familial and local support networks and was challenging in terms of the schooling of their eldest grandson, which was in a different locality and required Jane to get seven different buses. The process of becoming a kinship carer, which is already significantly emotional and often unanticipated, can also result in profound relational tension for these families and work against their efforts to keep their family together. Such processes are further compounded when access to adequate housing in localities is precarious and tenuous.

Anticipated welfare futures

The evidence presented in this chapter confirms that the everyday lives of families in the UK have been deeply affected by an array of cuts and reforms to state benefits and government support in the decade since 2010. These have had especially pernicious and disproportionate impacts on the everyday lives of families with children and families that were already socioeconomically disadvantaged (Jupp, 2017). Coupled with precarious employment and insecure housing, austerity policies have had the effect of deepening and worsening the financial hardships faced by families, limiting their access to basic amenities like food, housing and health (Jupp, 2017). As well as managing these everyday impacts, a pressing concern for these participants was how they would continue to provide financial and material support for their children in the long term, with the very real prospect of continued cuts to financial support.

For example, the inaccessibility of the labour market was further compounded by the complexities and increasingly punitive character of the welfare system. As a single father and primary caregiver for his adult disabled son, Matthew expressed concern about proposed changes to the welfare payments he and his son received, including his son's personal independence payments (Tarrant, 2018):

> 'With this Care Act,[1] if I don't work and I haven't got a job by then, you can't absorb these charges. You just can't do it. And I've got savings but they're not going to last forever. Because of the cuts, the austerity measures, [city] council have got – is it £74 million less in the next – last four years or something? It's a lot of money. So I don't know. So I've basically said to them, "I'll have no option but to be moving him to day care." Then you've probably taken away my options of working. A couple working could probably absorb these charges. A single person couldn't.'

Ridge (2009) highlights that families coping with a disabled child or adult need extra financial support because coping with disability and illness generates extra costs associated both with care and with disability.

Anticipated cuts to welfare are therefore an additional emotional burden on already financially and emotionally challenged families.

Looking forwards, Paul could only anticipate a future of further hardship: "It's just a hard life and the government's going to make it harder ... I mean financially, you know, to look after a child." Paul's reflection demonstrates how central financial vulnerabilities are in imagining future familial responsibilities, such that ideas, aspirations and worries about the future sit alongside one another. Matthew and Paul both anticipated that recession and austerity measures would further constrain their financial and familial futures (Hall, 2016a), while they themselves were providing huge savings to the state by providing care to young people experiencing often complex configurations of disadvantage. A clear paradox here is that while austerity is producing the conditions in which men are required to step in to provide care, this is a welfare context that also strips carers of their capabilities to do so effectively.

Concluding remarks

Where the previous chapter explored how, why and when men participate in family life, producing diverse familial arrangements, in this chapter the everyday processes and 'doing' of family life have been examined in conditions of a low income. These findings demonstrate the centrality of economic and financial vulnerabilities in the processes shaping men's family participation. Bringing the findings of this chapter into conversation with those in Chapter 5, it appears that the kinds of economic vulnerability produced are overridden by men's sense of responsibility to provide care for children, especially when those children's biographies are also shaped by deprivation processes and marked by trauma and loss. Nevertheless, the everyday financial and familial circumstances of these men's families illustrate how either a lack of state and government support in the form of welfare payments or an overzealous and punitive system of financial recuperation like the child maintenance system impacts on and heightens inequalities across households, worsens financial risk and increases vulnerability to poverty. Despite being commonly offset by a deep sense of family and community, the challenges of sustaining family life are paramount for these men.

Mirroring reflections elsewhere, when the family is viewed through an economic lens it is also possible to see how money and income infuse everyday family practices and strategies. As an inherently relational concept, provisioning captures the diverse variety of visible and invisible strategies that these men employ and is revealing of the material contexts in which they attempt to create a safe and supportive environment for their children. This includes the time-intensive and extensive strategies employed by those with care responsibilities that coalesce around the reconciliation of breadwinning and care. The focus here is less on how to be a good, involved father and occupied instead by how to navigate hardships and limited resources as a key aspect of family participation.

In parallel with previous research about low-income families experiencing deprivation (Emmel and Hughes, 2014), these narratives also reflect increased dependencies and engagements with a range of services to broker resources, in ways that can be either supportive or punitive. The precarity and financial vulnerability of these families means that they are often forced to live without basic resources, or to stretch money through budgeting. In some cases, they may also be required to draw on additional financial resources from wider family members including parents and partners, if such resources are available to them. How people manage poverty and income-based risks is therefore inherently relational and holds a significant place in the theorisation of families and intimate relationships in contexts of low income (Daly, 2018). The men who participated in the study, surprisingly, did not address explicit concerns about the implications of living in poverty in terms of their identities as men. This was perhaps mediated to some extent by their investments in their roles and responsibilities as caregivers. Thus, while the processes of provisioning and their financial relationships and negotiations with ex-partners are gendered, gender alone is not an adequate framework for explaining how and why they were able to support their families in low-income conditions.

The life-journey interviews also yielded data that spanned the macro-micro plane (Neale, 2019), revealing how the economic processes of recession and the political imposition of austerity formed significant social and historical contexts to the imagined futures of the participants and their families. The felt and personal impacts of austerity infused the everyday lives and anticipated futures of these men, lending further weight to observations that austerity constitutes a very personal crisis that both ruptures and fragments real and anticipated lifecourses (Hall, 2016a; 2019). While evidence suggests that the effects of austerity are most pernicious for young men (for example, McDowell, 2012), all the men in this study were impacted by welfare reforms and state-sanctioned requirements under the conditions of austerity to balance meaningful employment alongside their care responsibilities.

Men's family participation in low-income urban neighbourhoods

This final empirical chapter focuses on the experiences of men residing in a low-income locality in the city where the MPLC study was conducted. It reports on the ethnographic methods employed at a community centre based in an area of deprivation in the city. The centre was described as an important site of care and connectedness by the professionals who supported recruitment of participants to the study (see Chapter 4) and this was also confirmed by the men themselves. Ethnographic approaches have proven to be an effective means for identifying, engaging with and foregrounding the voices of ostensibly 'hard-to-reach' populations, including low-income families (Hemmerman, 2010) and disadvantaged and economically deprived fathers (Wissö, 2018). Indeed, despite policy and public alarmism about the pervasiveness of 'dad deprivation' (Ashe, 2014) and 'men deserts' in low-income localities across Britain, the centre was a space where the presence of men was observed, including visibly as fathers.

In accessing some of the more marginalised men in the city it was possible to observe how and why being a father or carer remains an important identity for men even when access to children may have been compromised or lost. The limits to men's family lives and relationships are also considered via the lens of their local engagement, social networks and community participation. With a proactive agenda towards supporting community members with their mental health, the community centre therefore became a key site for uncovering the lived experiences of diverse fathering in low-income contexts. As Bonner-Thompson and McDowell (2020) note, care itself has become much more precarious under the conditions of austerity, yet it has also enabled new and alternative spaces and practices of care to emerge (Power and Hall, 2017). As a locality-based policy and practice intervention creating opportunities for collective participation, the community centre was a key exemplar of this in the study.

The findings presented are further illustrative of the deprivations of context that shape men's identities and trajectories. This space was especially valuable to the older men, for whom connections to family had become more tenuous over time and were more transitory. I argue that knowledge of the locality and community-based resources is integral to an understanding of this group of participants and for the development of a rich, multi-layered understanding of the contexts shaping men's family participation in low-income contexts over time.

The reflections in this chapter are structured around an elaboration of the ethnographic methods employed to complement the interviews conducted with the core participants.

A contextual description of the locality

The community centre is situated in a low-income ward of the city. According to Middle Layer Super Output Area data, this is an area of the city with materially constrained conditions. Compared to the whole city, the locality recorded the second-highest proportion of men aged 30–49 who were single, and had the third-highest rate of recorded divorces. Data about whether these single men were fathers was not available, reflecting the national picture whereby father or 'daddy' data is meagre and does little to differentiate fathering status or relationships (Goldman and Burgess, 2017). In 2014, 5.9% of men in the locality had never worked (compared to a national average of 2.9%), and the ward was among the top five in the city with the highest proportion of NEET (not in employment, education or training) males aged 16–24. Between 2010 and 2012 the locality was also second only to one other area in the city in terms of rates of suicide for men aged 75 and under. It was also listed in the ten top-ranked Middle Layer Super Output Areas for high male hospital admission rates for self-harm between 2009 and 2011. In a report about the health of men in the city, a range of issues experienced by men residing in the locality were identified. For young men, having to leave the family home and sofa surfing were pertinent concerns (confirmed by the qualitative interviews and discussed in Chapter 6 of this book). Rates of long-term health conditions, unemployment, bullying and stress at work were also identified as high, and divorce and loss of contact with children were also key contributory factors to mental ill-health. Growing problems for older men were also attributed to a general lack of focused services for men in the city, compounding their poor social capital and networks and social isolation.[1]

The community centre therefore served an area of urban marginality that was physically, spatially and economically removed from wider society and thwarted by multiple deprivation. It is also a unique example of how communities adapt and develop solutions to mitigate the effects of material under-resource. The high levels of deprivation reported in the aggregate quantitative data were reflected in the narratives of the men residing in this locality, who were explicitly susceptible to the processes of marginalisation inherent in this place (see Emmel and Hughes, 2010). The locality, which is dominated by social housing tower blocks that house the highest proportion of single male residents in the city, is an archetypal 'sink estate', a label increasingly adopted in UK media and political discourse to describe public and social housing estates (Watt, 2020). Alongside discourses of parent blame, this language has been deployed as part of the wider ideological discourse used to justify austerity. Drawing on Wacquant's (2008a; Wacquant et al, 2014) influential framework, Watt (2020) suggests that the explicit labelling of 'sink estates' is a form of 'territorial stigmatisation', a major vector of advanced urban marginality. As I argue with colleagues elsewhere (Ward et al, 2017; Tarrant and Hughes, 2020), responsibility for poverty and the stigmatisation of locality often accrues to the people who live there, and they become vilified on the basis of class- and race-based inequalities and the 'blemish of place' (Wacquant, 2008b). In this process, poverty is 'de-contextualised and individualised, and urban areas and neighbourhoods, become "spatially tainted" through their links to a range of social problems' (Crossley, 2017 cited by Tarrant and Hughes, 2020: 292). In this chapter, the processes of marginalisation that contour the biographies of these men, men who are themselves stigmatised as absent fathers, shirkers and undeserving, are examined in the context of an equally and problematically stigmatised place.

Immersion in life at the community centre

As noted in Chapter 4, I was alerted to the important work of the community centre by one of the study partners. I was put in contact with the manager, Gavin (a pseudonym), whom I visited to learn more about the community-building work they were doing and how they were engaging with and supporting men in the locality. Gavin expressed an interest in the research because much of his work had been centred on creating a supportive and caring environment for men in the locality, where, as confirmed by quantitative data, high rates of suicide among middle-aged men had been observed as a pressing problem, injecting a palpable atmosphere of unease into the locality. These suicides were mentioned several times, often unprompted, both by Gavin and in informal conversations with community centre attendees:

Jed: The flats need cutting down a bit. Make them four flats. Not sixteen floors. People do jump out of those flats. That is sad.

Bill: You hear it all the time. 'Have you heard such and such has died?'... there's quite a lot of single guys.

Bill's observation that predominantly single men lived in the towers, chimed with that of the housing manager, whose observations of successive housing policies were discussed in Chapter 4. She argued that changes in housing policy were having observable impacts on older, single men by enforcing their social isolation. In an interview with Graham, age 45, one of the centre regulars whom I got to know well and who was also one of the 26 men comprising the core participant group, he remarked:

> 'There's a lot of drug dealers around here, car robbers, you can't leave one sock outside, that's how bad it is ... the flats, people are always jumping out of them. There have been a couple of deaths round here ... only one person I know jumped out of that [points to tower through the window]. [Friend at the centre] knows him too ... I can't remember when, about two years ago now? [Friend at the centre]'s mate jumped out of that flat, this one here. Jumped out of that window. Yes, it's not nice, keep yourself to yourself, you're okay.'

The findings in this locality support long-standing findings in research about suicide indicating that completed male suicide rates are typically three to four times higher among men than women (Jordan and Chandler, 2019). High suicide rates in men are often conflated with the 'crisis of masculinity', reinforcing problematic gender politics (Jordan and Chandler, 2019) and obscuring class-based inequalities in the emphasis on gender. Notably in this study, while the participants theorised that single men in the locality were especially vulnerable to suicide because they had become increasingly socially isolated due to successive housing policy and the violence of place, this was just one part of the story. As part of a broader interest in men's participation in low-income contexts I determined that it was important to learn more about why this was happening, as a route to accessing accounts of men's biographies and their social and relational lives, in this case, in a specific context of urban marginality and deprivation.

Gavin confirmed that I could spend some time at the centre so I could get to know people and observe its rhythms. The community centre was a dynamic space, including a community shop and cafe, a residents' association, housing surgery, food bank and healthy-living network. To support and engage residents in the locality, the centre had a varied programme of weekly activities designed to provide a social security net, to support well-being and to increase employability for all residents. The activities included support groups, voluntary opportunities (including a gardening group and positive communication group), exercise groups (including Zumba classes) and the urban walk for men (led by another of the project partners, see Chapter 4). On their own initiative, several of the men had also started up their own rock band and were excited by their most recent plans to establish an open mic poetry night. The community centre was also frequented by professionals from the council and other welfare and family support agencies who visited to provide advice or deliver support clinics.

After only a very short period of immersion it became clear that the centre was a significant space of local engagement and belonging and was pivotal to the maintenance of the social fabric of the community, providing essential social and material supports. I spent many hours at the community centre between August 2015 and August 2016, observing the comings and goings, the interactions, eating food from the cafe and meeting the many men, women and children it supported. Reflecting the population profile described by the quantitative data, the centre was attended by men and women of all age groups, as well as by families, including young parents and grandparents. On one occasion I got into conversation with a heavily pregnant young teenage mum and her mother, who had dropped in to have a rest and a cup of tea before heading back home from the city centre, which was just over a mile away. On another, when a housing officer from the council had arrived to provide his fortnightly open clinic where residents could express or attempt to resolve concerns about their housing issues, I witnessed an angry exchange. An older male resident who had a young child in a buggy was expressing a clear sense of powerlessness in relation to the lack of opportunity available to him to resolve his housing problems. He could be visibly heard lamenting both the council and the government, who he felt were not responding to or listening to him. In passing, another man said, "it's good to come here if you need anything like aftershave". Others visited to socialise, purchase food, which was being served cheaply at the café, and to access the small food bank and the IT equipment which was available for use to find employment opportunities. This was a vital space for community cohesion, the acquisition of resources and social support.

Several of the men I met and saw regularly at the centre and on the two urban walks that I joined agreed to participate in interviews for the study. I was able to interview six men initially: Graham, age 45, a non-resident father with learning difficulties, whose three children had been removed for adoption at birth; Lewis, who was not a biological father but described multiple caring responsibilities across his lifecourse, including for siblings, nieces and nephews; Alan, a grandfather, step-father and ex-carer for his elderly father; Marvin, a 61-year-old grandfather and step-father; and Andy and Dean, the two dads who visited the centre together. Andy explained that he had two daughters, the first with whom he had lost touch, and a teenage daughter who stayed with him in his small flat every other week. He slept on the couch when his daughter stayed because his flat was too small to accommodate them both. He was addicted to drugs but expressed a desire to get clean for the sake of his daughter. His friend Dean, who had one of his young sons with him during the interview, was a father to four children and was still resident and living with the mother of his children. He was also unemployed.

Collectively, these men's family biographies were the most fraught of the core participant group. They expressed a range of disadvantages and their stories of fatherhood and fathering represented the most tenuous among the participants I spoke to. The men responded to their material circumstances in different ways but all described histories of poverty and deprivation, chaotic family backgrounds, anger and histories of violence (through gang-based behaviours and towards female partners), addictions and disconnection both from secure employment and personal relationships. For these participants, limited employment opportunities, engagements in the informal economy (for example, dealing drugs, exchanging goods), poor mental health and the loss of partners and access to children isolated them and led to mental ill-health and linked dependencies on alcohol and other stimulants. Nevertheless, they invested heavily in their family identities, and were keen to present themselves as 'good fathers'. Andy and Dean were exemplars of this. These were the same two men that I had observed popping into the centre to pick up the paint brushes so that Dean could paint his child's bedroom. They explained that they were good friends and that Andy was helping Dean with his decorating. Notably, they had very different backgrounds, caring arrangements and strategies for presenting good fatherhood. While they both reflected on how important fatherhood was to them, Andy explained how his ongoing addiction to heroin mitigated against his efforts to be regularly involved in his daughter's life. Dean was more careful to explain that he was not addicted to drugs but that he did use with Andy recreationally when he was not responsible for the children (that is, when his wife was caring for them). They both agreed that being a father is important, but Andy expressed difficulty in managing his addiction, which became established in his adolescent years:

Andy: It's brilliant being a dad, god yeah course it is, it's best thing int' world …
Dean: [overlapping] best thing in the world.
Andy: Best thing int' world, yeah, but, like a dick 'ed, I still carry on you know what I mean? I told meself so many times like I won't gonna do this, I won't gonna do that and yet I come out.

The narratives of Andy and Dean indicate the shared centrality of fatherhood as a generational identity in men even in the most precarious of circumstances. However, in contrast to most of the MPLC participants who were identified through different support organisations (and whose narratives are analysed in Chapters 5 and 6), and for more resourced men who are primary caregivers and become isolated because they are fathers (for example, Richards Solomon, 2017), these men were much more disconnected from their family lives and described limited sets of interdependencies, producing periods of social isolation. Their familial and social circumstances therefore reflected the material realities and the constraints of this locality, where they had lived for most of their lives. Opportunities for caregiving and familial connection were much more fragile and, while implicit, it was this disconnection, both from a secure family life and employment, that had brought them to the centre.

Notwithstanding these chaotic and insecure trajectories, for these participants, the community centre was a significant space of care and personal transformation; a lifeline in a world of violence and social isolation. Lewis, age 38, who was receiving £120 a week in social security payments, explained what he did at the centre and why it was so vital to him. When prompted, he also noted the alternatives if it were not there:

Lewis: I came here to start with cleaning outside. It needed doing. I was doing it voluntary … I've been doing bits and bobs since. Cleaning. Wiping sides down. Mopping.

Sweeping up leaves. Scraping pavements. Emptying the bin. Gardening. Carrying things. Bits of laundry.

Anna: What would you be doing if this wasn't here?

Lewis: Smoking weed and kicking back and relaxing. Or in the bookies.

Perhaps one of the more memorable narrative reflections about the value and significance of the centre that illustrated this finding effectively was articulated during an interview with Graham, age 45 (see Figure 7.1). His life journey and narrative are presented here as an exemplar of the kinds of trajectories that were being described by the participants at the centre.

Graham was unemployed and received £140 a fortnight in welfare payments. He had learning difficulties but he was outgoing and well known at the community centre, which was near his home in one of the nearby tower blocks. He was also one of the quickest to talk to me and engage with the research. As demonstrated by the quote presented, he described how the mechanisms for survival in his locality had changed for him over time. Where he once engaged in violent behaviour (as a gang member and in his relationship with the mother of his children), he now engaged in community life at the community centre. Graham linked his own expressions of anger and violence to a range of adverse experiences in his upbringing and familial biography, in which he witnessed his father being violent towards his mother, leading to social services intervention. Taking his father's violence and his experience in care as a starting point, it was also possible to piece together aspects of his life journey as shaped by ongoing marginalisation and a longer history of connection to the locality. This included engagements in violence as part of a local gang in the area, associated anger issues, the perpetration of domestic violence himself, dependence on alcohol and, eventually, the loss of his wife and four children, who were in care. Each of these factors is indicative of when men are much too present in family contexts and when their involvement in the lives of children and mothers is highly disruptive and problematic (Roy et al, 2015). I present Graham's experience as part of an extended and reconstructed narrative from his interviews. Reflecting on his own father first:

Graham: He kept going out drinking, kept on gambling and kept on going, dating women and then coming back drunk and hitting me mam, like hitting his wife and all that kind of thing. So, that went wrong. We then got put into care and then my mam got asked to choose him or the kids. So she ...

Figure 7.1: Going to the community centre

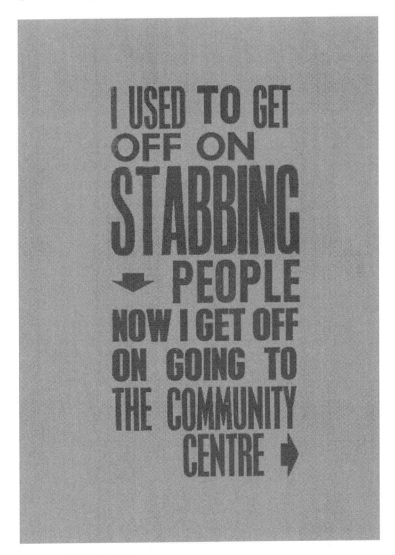

Source: © Katie Smith 2017

Anna:	Oh, by Social Services is this?
Graham:	Yeah. So she picked us, she dumped him and went, bye, go. So, she did everything for us. She did the cooking, washing, taking us out to parks, taking us out places like shops, getting our eyes tested, new shoes, cafes, holidays, like Butlins, seaside towns, she took us everywhere.

I were part of a gang. We went round robbing houses, nicking cars and taking drugs, taking gas, glue, setting fire to people's cars, setting fire to people's houses. And then when I got older I messed around, got messing with another lad that were like knee-capping people for money and all that kind of thing ... taking things out of shops and doing that he were – they were doing rackets that they shouldn't be, knee-capping for money and I thought, no, better give up, too dodgy and I don't want to end up in prison.

I have a bad temper too. Every time people kept talking to me I kept walking up to them and punching them in the face. My ex-wife, Poppy, pointed that out, about my temper. Because like it never bothered me at first 'til I got my two – Poppy, my wife, ex-wife, and then my temper kept coming out on her and I think, why we lost our kids because I was drinking. Because I must have a bit of my dad's side or something, and I were drinking. I were – well, Poppy my ex-wife, and I didn't work, I was signing on and I took it out on her.

To Graham as an older man in the locality, the centre provided a source of friendship, belonging and the ability to acquire key resources and skills in ways that he had been unable to earlier in his life. It also enabled him to address and understand the anger and violence that ultimately resulted in him losing his wife and children.

The value of the centre as a place for enabling a positive turning point and change was an experience shared by Will, too. He was a 44-year-old father of four, who had recently separated from his wife and become a non-resident father. He explained that the death of his father when he was 12 years old was formative and deeply affected him and his perception of his life, because it had left him without a father figure. His mother was unable to care for him properly and he had lost his way. He made his own breakfast, lunch and tea and felt isolated because he didn't have the money to do the things his friends were able to do. Will became a teenage father when he was 18 and his children's mother, now his ex-wife, was 16.

Will attended the community centre because he had become isolated since the breakdown of his marriage, the loss of access to his children and because of a number of other disruptive life-altering events: the loss of his job following accusations that he had stolen from the company he was working for, and allegations of sexual abuse within his family. His son, Jamie, who had learning difficulties, had been arrested on suspicion of the sexual assault of one of his younger brothers. The police and social services had become involved because of the risk posed to the younger children. This incident had caused problems within the wider family unit and led to the eventual breakdown of Will's marriage and loss of his children. Jamie was cleared of the assault, but social services had wanted Jamie to get a house of his own. Will didn't agree with this decision because, although Jamie was 16, he had a mental age of 11. This had resulted in Will getting angry and frustrated with social services and he was accused of being abusive towards them and his ex-partner. He then explained that he had had to choose between his wife and his kids because he was perceived as a threat to his children. Each of these processes had triggered a period of homelessness. The divorce process and an issue with over-claiming child benefit when the two younger children were in foster care meant that, between them, Will and his ex-wife were also £4,000 in debt.

This had led to an emotional breakdown, where Will explained, he lost his way. He became manic-depressive and suicidal and was given a prison sentence for breaking a restraining order against him for going too close to his ex-wife. Will was attending the community centre because he wanted to forget about this history and focus on himself. As a newcomer, he was apprehensive about the place and the people, but he said, 'in some respects this community centre has become a bit of a sanctuary'. It helped him to get out of his flat, which he described as small and mouldy. He had walked for 1 hour and 20 minutes to attend on the day of the interview because he had seen a poster advertising a music session. His probation officer had also signposted it to him.

In exploring these men's life journeys and biographies it was clear that, over time, spaces like the community centre took on a renewed significance and, for some, offered the companionship and resources required to survive as an older man in low-income localities. It is important to note here that these trajectories are not presented to further stigmatise these men or the locality, which, as the community centre provision demonstrates, are also spaces where care and community can flourish. These narratives are presented instead to demonstrate the material realities of the participants in ways that shift blame from participants for their familial absence, while also acknowledging their ongoing capacity to act.

Many of the men at the centre also demonstrated their commitment to investing in the community as a kind of reparation for past problems. For example attendance at the community centre had a reciprocal character and engendered an ethos of exchange in the participants.

It was not only a space for accessing and receiving support; it also provided opportunities for volunteering, local investment and giving back to the community. Marvin and Lewis explain:

Marvin: The people in it [the community centre] are important. It's what I can do for the centre rather than what it can do for me ... There's a task force for anyone disabled or unable to do their own decorating or jobs around the house. Gardens or whatever. If you have a council house you are responsible for the maintenance of the garden. That worries people. So we go out and do that.

Lewis: With me being unemployed with nothing to do this place has been a godsend. I volunteer two days a week. And I love it. It gets me out the house.

Capturing locality-based resources: walking photovoice

I spent several months immersing myself at the community centre, observing the comings and goings, the value of the space for those who attended, and engaging with attendees to learn more about the locality and how it was experienced by marginalised men and local families. Towards the end of the fieldwork period an opportunity arose to use cameras that I purchased for the study for the purposes of photovoice (Tarrant and Hughes, 2020), for a walking activity with members of the centre. The manager Gavin was planning a celebratory event in June 2016 and, in advance of the event, he planned to record some audio from the locality with a small group to develop a soundscape. I asked him if I could join them and bring the cameras with me. The images taken by the participants would support insights into the locality and into participant experience, and I offered the images to be presented at the celebratory events.

I describe this method as 'walking photovoice' because it combined elements of visual urban ethnography and biographical walking methods. Informed by a rich, emerging body of debate concerning the value of walking and visual methods (for example, Fink and Lomax, 2014; Delgado, 2015; McCulloch, 2018; O'Neill and Roberts, 2019), walking photovoice involved participant-led walking interviews combined with photography and guided conversations. The participants were instructed to document and explain what they considered to be significant about their locality, and revealed fascinating insights about what it was like to be a man residing in this area of the city, including the opportunities and constraints for participation. The method produced rich, in-depth insights about the social and relational dynamics of men's lives in low-income contexts and thus responded to my research questions. The activity was conducted with five participants; Will, Graham and Richard (the latter whom I had seen at the centre several times but had not spoken to before), Jodie, a young mother who was with her young daughter, and her friend, Leanne. This method appealed to me, a social geographer by background, with its potential to reveal these men's carescapes (Bowlby et al, 2010) and the community-based resources and networks that were so significant in providing them with material supports hitherto missing in their earlier lifecourses. Such questions and evidence were also rendered especially significant in a context of austerity, where resources are being systematically stripped back and are increasingly scarce.

Via this method, we collaboratively explored the local urban landscape, prompting additional reflections about the participants' biographies, including personal and relational factors; the rhythms and temporalities of the locality; and insights into what I conceptualise as urban 'spaces of care'. The method further supported in-depth exploration of the role of the community centre and locality as a key context in the shaping of men's care responsibilities, experiences and citizenship. Perhaps unsurprisingly, the community centre was a focal point for the images produced and was described as one of the key places that the participants liked most. In the follow-up interviews, which took place in the centre, other attendees came over and looked through and commented on the images, describing what they liked about the locality and what they valued about the community centre space. One of the male participants whom I had not met before explained:

'Everybody from round here are lovely. It's nice. It's [the locality] always had a bad reputation ... There's a lot of nice people here. Lot of help.

'They have a few outlets. They bend over backwards to help you. With mental health it really helps ... I work on loads of music projects. But don't put me in front of a microphone. Two weeks ago, I was doing a workshop and I was a backing singer to the girls here. ... I suppose the friendship aspect to it is important. And nobody is judging you. It's human nature to talk about something.'

Lots of the images taken depicted well-kept gardens on the estate. When asked to comment on this afterwards, tower block resident Richard noted the limited opportunities available for using and working in the garden space outside the tower block:

'I just like people who look after their gardens. It would be nice if councils spent a bit more money. Where I live, that bit of grass round our blocks is virtually our garden. Can't go out to the garden because they won't let us. Effectively that bit of grass is our garden. I'd like to see more flowers.'

The prison and tower blocks featured more heavily in aspects of the place that were considered less positive. The prison in particular was described as being fed in observable cycles by men residing in the locality. The local pharmacy and betting shops also featured heavily in the images, and the participants explained that these were the only other places left in the locality for men to socialise, congregate and access health services. The participants were astute observers of social change in the locality, remarking on processes of urban change. Marvin, who was an ex-biker, described the heartbreak he experienced when his home was knocked down during the process of slum clearance. Demonstrating a clear attachment to place he said:

'Quite a few of us lived in derelict houses because at that time there was slum clearance, you see. The old back-to-back terraces. They did it all over [city]. Some parts of [city] are unrecognisable now. I used to have dreams about it. Because I hated them knocking the houses down. I'd grown up with them. I loved them. My grandparents lived in them. My parents in theirs. All that, you know? I thought what are you doing knocking my world down? No consideration at all. It was we're going to bulldoze you out the way. Way it seemed like to me.'

Several of the participants were also notably witnessing the erosion of spaces for sociability in the area. The gambling shops featured prominently in the photovoice images and were identified as spaces of change, where men now congregate in lieu of an absence of local pubs. Referring directly to an image of the gambling shops (not included, to protect the identity of the locality), Graham said:

'A lot of pubs and clubs have shut down ... lot of the socialising places have closed down.
   This one [pointing to one of the images] was like of the gambling place. Trying to change addictions and stuff. Quite a lot of people abuse it. Some of them have got addictions. It's something that we'd want to change.'

The tower blocks overlooking the community centre were a central focal point of the images and were symbolic of both the identity of the locality and the social problems inherent to it. In reference to the image depicted in Figure 7.2, the young mother who participated in the walking photovoice even stated: "It's [locality]. The towers there. Move the towers it wouldn't be [locality]."

Mirroring existing research with low-income families living in deprived neighbourhoods (Ridge, 2009), the participants also expressed concerns about the range of social problems that they witnessed around the housing blocks and on the streets where they lived, including drug use, prostitution and violence. In the follow-up interview after the walking photovoice activity the participants explained that they regularly observed drug taking and prostitution in the entrance to the flats, and in some cases this meant that they would not invite their parents and other family members to visit, or their families would refuse to visit them. In explaining why the locality is viewed as a place that is *not for families*, Richard noted:

'There was a bloke shouting outside our flats. He didn't have a fob to get in. It's about one o'clock in the morning. A lad leaned out and asked him to keep it down, kids are in bed.

Figure 7.2: The towers; taken during the walking photovoice

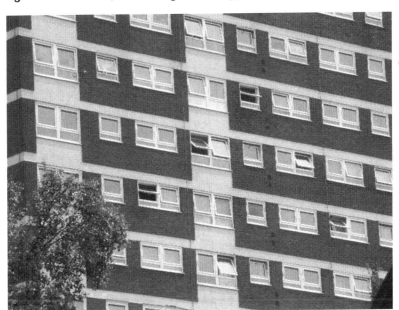

Source: © Anna Tarrant 2016

And the guy turned around and asked him what he was doing here living with kids. It's a shithole. Carried on shouting. People in my block come in and wee in the lift. And they live there. I know animals that don't do that. It's embarrassing. I don't want my mum or family to come and see me. My mum has been greeted by a prostitute. My mum is worldly and knows what's what. But I don't want her to see that.'

Graham also described that he often picked up used needles if he saw them on the streets, to ensure that local children would not pick them up. He commented that he had a pile of five of them on the top of his shelf at home; the police showed no interest in disposing of them and the doctor's surgery wouldn't take them, he commented.

The locality itself was also described as particularly dangerous to navigate for young men, reflecting how experiences of the locality were interpreted by residents as gendered experiences that were also devoid of connection and care (Figure 7.3):

Anna: What does it mean to be a man around here?
Jodie: You've got to be in gangs.
Leanne: When you are female, they don't feel like they have to pull you into it. We could walk around any time we wanted. Not get hassled. If guys do it they have

Figure 7.3: Being a man in the locality; taken during the walking photovoice

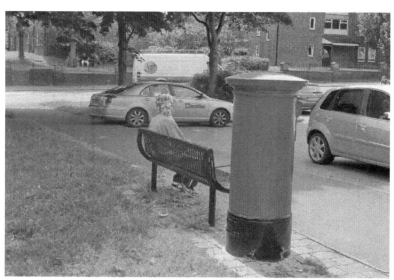

Source: © Anna Tarrant 2016

to be careful at nights. My first boyfriend. He went
down to shop and it got dark. It took him a while
but I got worried. If I had gone and took me a while,
I wouldn't have worried.

As is noted elsewhere, drawing on a large and established academic
literature that is empirically based on young men who reside in deprived
post-industrial localities (Ward et al, 2017), local neighbourhoods, gang
involvement and poor employment prospects play a key role in forming
and shaping the masculine identities, performances and transitions of
young, urban, working-class men. In a service economy characterised
by deindustrialisation where young, working-class men have become
disadvantaged in their search for employment, for example, young men
may conform to versions of 'protest' masculinity. Involvement in urban
unrest may be a typical response (McDowell et al, 2014). Anomic forms
of protest masculinity (Walker, 2006) may constitute acts of antisocial
behaviour in public spaces, including 'aggression, violence, physicality,
substance misuse, drinking large amounts of alcohol and excessive
heterosexuality and homophobic language' (Ward et al, 2017: 800).

However, protest masculinity must be understood in context as an
outcome of marginalisation, either from economic resources or from
racial signifiers (Majors, 1998; hooks, 2004). Connell (1995) was the
first to inject a class analysis, derived from concepts of 'masculine
protest' and 'compulsory masculinity' developed by Parsons (1954),
to describe these behaviours. It is also worth noting here that more
fluid performative masculinities have been identified among young,
white, working-class men, linked to a combined commitment to a
search for employment and domestic respectability (McDowell et al,
2014). Moreover, while gangs and young people's associated practices
are often spectacularised and misunderstood as violent, the collective
and risk-taking behaviours of young people are often quite banal,
routinised (Bengtsson and Ravn, 2019) and involve a lot of hanging
about (Fraser, 2015). Gangs can therefore be an important source of
collective identity and relationality that many young men are less likely
to experience in family contexts after a certain age.

Ashe (2014: 656) also argues that conditions of economic
marginalisation have differential impacts on young men and women,
suggesting that 'they shape masculinities and femininities (Campbell,
1993), and mediate how protest, grievance and resistance are both
generated and expressed'. While there are opportunities for increased
fluidity in performances of masculinities, such as those that in this
locality were being enabled through the support of the community

centre, the 'fixing mechanisms that limit the fluidity of identities' (Connell, 2001: 8), namely the structural contexts in which masculinities are performed, are essential for developing sociological explanation of men's experiences in deprived post-industrial economies and localities (see also Heward, 1996; Ward et al, 2017). It appears that younger and older men have different opportunities and trajectories available to them in this locality, with young men building up forms of support in the violent context of local gangs while older men seek new connections and collective forms of participation at the community centre.

Despite attention to the stigma attached to the locality and its social problems, which rendered it unsafe for family life and for individuals along gendered dimensions, later in the discussions the community centre with its walled communal garden was described as a haven for families because it provided a safe space for children to play, as well as opportunities for personal growth. Leanne, who took several photographs of the garden explained:

> 'I was so shy when I first came here. I haven't shut up since. I don't get to go out with my brothers because we live on a dangerous estate. And they can come to the centre and sit out and stuff. And play football. They are not going to run off anywhere because there are people to watch them.'

In evidence were the ways in which both caring and protest masculinities coexist in this space. In these ways, the walking photovoice activity countered some of the conventional wisdoms of low-income localities, demonstrating what is valued about these places, alongside their problems. It was also revealing of some of the processes that may isolate men from their family contexts and identities.

Concluding remarks

A very different story of men's family participation has been explored in this chapter. The narratives of these men reveal the limits to family participation and fathering when processes and mechanisms of deprivation and poverty are so entrenched that they lead to the breakdown and disconnection of men's family relationships across the lifecourse producing social isolation. The rationale and methodological approaches developed to research the relational and social character of low-income life for men in this specific area of urban marginality and deprivation were also elaborated. Alerted by the MPLC stakeholders to the vital work of the community centre in facilitating social connections (see Chapter 4), it was possible to access accounts of marginalised fatherhoods and non-familial caregiving in a socioeconomic and geographic context where men are much less materially resourced. The ethnography of the community centre, including the walking photovoice activity and complementary semi-structured and informal interviews, revealed some of the place-based and 'entangled inequalities' (Fluri and Peidalue, 2017) that these marginalised men experience and negotiate across the lifecourse, including how the enduring character of vulnerability and marginalisation impinges on family connections, social networks and relations.

Significantly, the community centre was a vital local policy intervention providing opportunities for men to repair social connections and establish new forms of participation as citizens, for example, through their voluntary work. This was therefore a transformative space that produced opportunities for men to develop relational networks outside of the family and in ways that enabled them to sustain and manage their lives in the context of wider structural inequalities and socioeconomic change. As the cases of Graham and Will illustrate, it supported men to transition to alternative masculinities in their adult lives in ways that rejected the practices of violence and hyper-masculinity that were, and still are, typically required of men to navigate and survive the locality. Via an analysis of the empirical accounts of men of different ages and at different stages of the lifecourse, the findings and interpretations presented in this chapter therefore advance understandings of the relationships between masculinities, class and place (for example, Ward et al, 2017) and their longitudinal character and implications. They also evidence the value of a radical reimaging of marginality as 'openness' in which empowerment processes and practices of caring masculinities might be encouraged to flourish for 'men in the margin' (Elliott, 2020) and in marginal spaces and localities through targeted policy support.

Researching across age groups in this space also reflected the methodological design of MPLC, enabling analysis both within the cases and across the cases more generally. Graham's insights about being a gang member in his younger days for example were confirmed by the young mothers who participated in the walking photovoice. They verify, alongside a broad academic literature identifying the same (for example, Anderson, 1999; Deuchar, 2009; Gunter and Watt, 2009; Fraser, 2015), that gang participation is a key contextual feature of young, working-class men's trajectories to adulthood and survival in post-industrial localities like this one. Advancing evidence in the existing academic literature, Graham's account also provides rare insight into the mechanisms for disengagement from gangs and desistence from crime. In Graham's case the essential role of the community centre was highlighted in producing a turning point away from the perpetration of violence and from the structural and performative violence of the locality.

Will's account as a 44-year-old father who had been a young father himself and whose parenting identity and journey remained central to his self-narrative may also be considered a prospective account of young fathers' long-term trajectories through marginalisation into adulthood. In researching men of different ages, MPLC enabled analysis across generations and consideration of whether Will's case might be deemed what we call a 'data proxy' for other young fathers (Tarrant and Hughes, 2019). This is not to suggest that longer-term trajectories for young fathers in similar localities will always be the same. Rather, the longer-term processes of marginalisation, including insecure employment, the pressures of raising multiple children (including some who have additional support needs) and the increasing regulation of family life by formal agencies like social services may increase men's risk and vulnerability to social isolation and loss of familial connection in the long term.

Finally, while the participants illustrated some of the social problems that characterised the locality, significantly, the walking photovoice enabled counter narratives of this stigmatised place to emerge. Processes of deprivation and the stigmatisation of localities that were constructed by the participants as *not for families* can impinge on family lives and personal connections. However, in this context, the community centre was a valued space for community, belonging and support that was hitherto absent for some men. Notably, for example, many of the participants considered it to be a haven or sanctuary, providing opportunities for communication, connection and participation that were otherwise hard to find in the locality. Spaces like these are increasingly under threat of closure under the conditions of austerity, yet, as these findings illustrate, they are essential for enabling communities and individuals to adapt and to resist the vulnerabilities that constitute their individual biographies and contexts. These findings contribute further evidence about how men's issues are shaped within specific contexts and localised cultures (Ward et al, 2017), both over time and across the lifecourse. The essential need to account for the structural and spatial inequalities and processes that shape men's life trajectories and biographies of blemished places are also highlighted, in ways that address societal stigmatisation and individualised explanations of poverty, as well as the unfolding of events and processes that render men absent in particular family and policy contexts.

8

Conclusion: Men's family participation in low-income contexts

Fathering and Poverty both connects with and contributes to, ongoing public and policy debates and interdisciplinary scholarship about pressing and intersecting societal discussions and debates. These include men, masculinities and fatherhood; gender and care; and the lived experiences of family poverty. Taking forward ideas about fathering, families and poverty in new ways that have implications for practice and policy, this chapter confirms the overall thesis for the book. It argues that in a context of social ambivalence about men as carers, men with caring responsibilities remain highly isolated and welfare and market provision for 'caring masculinities' is being neither produced nor sustained.

In evidencing this argument and elaborating these advances, the key conclusions from the MPLC study are summarised to foreground the dynamic, relational, intersectional and context-specific character of men's experiences of low-income family life and caregiving across the lifecourse. This necessarily more complicated view of men and their participation in low-income families and contexts supports a more detailed understanding of the complex and evolving relationship between fathers, poverty, families and policy. I also re-emphasise that the realities of family and fathering for men in low-income contexts are often rendered invisible in research despite their heightened visibility in policy and public arenas.

It is important to acknowledge here that in bringing men's family participation in low-income families to the fore, the intention is not to generalise about the diverse and divergent trajectories and biographies of men in low-income families. Similarly, the arguments made are not offered to deny when some men are absent from households and family contexts. Indeed, Chapter 1 presents statistical evidence of father absence from households caused by change in family structures and within couple relationships. Chapter 7 also considers some of the mechanisms and processes that produce men's familial absence, highlighting where men are sometimes present in problematic ways as well. However, qualitative accounts of the meaning and experience of family for men, alongside evidence of some of the vital contributions that men make in low-income family contexts, are explored here in a societal context where they are typically obscured, broadly stigmatised and men are deprived both of recognition of their capabilities to care and of recognition of the value and significance of their family identities.

The chapter begins by recapping the MPLC study on which the advances in this book are based. The conceptualisation of family participation is then elaborated, followed by attention to the way in which low-income contexts impinge on men's efforts towards their families. These sections of the chapter build an argument that men's care practices and the doing of kinship are varied, change over time and are influenced by their biographies, interdependencies and situation in a web of privileges and inequalities. The chapter concludes with implications for policy and practice and suggests future directions for research.

The contributions of MPLC

Offering a robust contribution to existing debates, which often delineate between men's absence and presence as fathers, the conclusions presented in this chapter are based on extensive and detailed fieldwork, analysis and engagement with existing data and literature. The MPLC fieldwork had explicit connections to, and built out of, empirical engagement with legacy data that had captured the social and relational worlds of men in low-income families over an extended 12-year period (Emmel and Hughes 2014; Neale et al, 2015). Detailed analysis of the relationships between fathering, poverty and policy had not been explicitly conducted using data from these studies. In engaging with this data, a unique qualitative longitudinal approach was employed, that analytically connected the findings of the IGE and FYF studies with new empirical data (Tarrant, 2017; Tarrant and Hughes, 2019). The longitudinal accretion of data from these studies and extended engagement with a whole landscape of evidence, extended the possibilities of drawing across a wider body of evidence in support of discussions about the key thematic areas.

While theoretically relevant snippets of the IGE and FYF data feature in the introductory chapter and were referred to when relevant, the overall focus of this book has been the new empirical findings generated. This data, much of which builds incrementally from these original studies (i.e., through interviews with young fathers and male kinship carers) constitutes additional and extended evidence of the life journeys of men with diverse familial arrangements and generational identities. Producing multiple perspectives, these were also combined with interviews with professionals who had a remit to support men, as well as ethnographic and participatory methods that explored men's orientations towards their care roles and responsibilities in low-income families and localities. These combined sets of data constitute a more robust and longitudinal evidence base, built on data histories of men's family lives in low-income contexts.

As well as engaging longitudinally with these data histories, the design of MPLC was relatively rare in seeking to uncover the caring responsibilities of men in different generational positions who occupy diverse father and/or father like relationships in what might be called 'non-conventional' or non-normative family contexts (Finch, 2007). Where existing research has engaged with questions of men and care it often dwells on biological fathers as a particular generational and familial position. The unique and important contribution of MPLC, and therefore of this book, is the intergenerational and multi-generational character of the participant group. Alongside new empirical accounts of recognised marginalised fatherhoods like young and lone fatherhoods, MPLC generated insights about the lives of older men, which, via prospective and retrospective accounts, revealed the longitudinal processes that lead to informal and state-ratified practices of kinship care later in life. Men's experiences of kinship care are less understood in the empirical emphasis on either women's experiences as carers or on younger fathers, who are most likely to be recognised as marginalised by their age and generational position.

Overall, the study methods supported an in-depth examination of men's pathways to care, their everyday caring practices and the doing of kinship, the meanings they ascribe to their responsibilities and reflections on their engagements with services and welfare agencies. Foregrounding men's perspectives, the study findings further determined the relational dynamics of men's lives and diverse trajectories, the patterning and everyday nature of their care responsibilities, the processes that produce household absence and involvement over time and their situatedness in a complex network of interdependencies both longitudinally and generationally.

The study has also prompted a robust critique of the ways in which men in low-income contexts are represented and understood in current policy and practice contexts, addressing the questions of how and why men in low-income families so often continue to evoke moral panic (Cohen, 2002) and condemnation in the popular and policy imaginary (also see Neale and Davies, 2016). Indeed, the opening chapters of this book began to shed critical light on dominant policy and practice framings of fathers residing in low-income localities and family contexts as a starting point for raising a more reflective set of questions around the processes producing the (in)visibilities of men in such contexts. The problematic gendered and classed assumptions that pervade contemporary public and political commentary point to individualised problems with men and families. The 'problem' of boys has been identified, ostensibly caused by the absence of men and fathers in the UK's poorest localities and communities and other social institutions. Crisis rhetoric that is embedded in policy and practice emphasises intergenerational cycles of disadvantage where cultures of deprivation and parenting deficit are assumed to pass down the generations raising concerns about the impact of absent fatherhood and fatherless societies on the future adult male identities of boys. As a result, positive male role models in key institutions are often posed as a solution.

Historical scholarship (which is charted in Chapter 2) further indicates that dominant methodologies and theoretical histories have also long been a component of the processes that preclude empirical consideration of men's subjective experiences of, and marginalisation from, family life, explaining why, in part, they have rarely been subject to critique or more detailed examination. Through the continued omission of men's voices, lived experiences and accounts of family life, academic scholarship has contributed, perhaps inadvertently, to the perpetuation of pessimistic stereotypes and discourses that accrue to fathers (both biological and social) residing in working-class and low-income families and localities. Recent developments in social-historical research are beginning to recover and reintegrate men back into the family and critique their historic marginalisation from families. This body of work demonstrates that men have always been embedded in family contexts and introduces some caution that their marginal status in the family might be more reflective of ideology, culture and the analytical lenses through which men's experiences are apprehended, rather than reflective of the empirical and material realities of families. These arguments suggest that the policy rhetoric of 'absent fathers', a moral narrative, is problematic because it atomises men and fails to account for the diverse sets of interdependencies in which men are embedded.

Drawing distinct parallels with the arguments of social historical research but using contemporary data and evidence, MPLC directly addressed assumptions of the peripheral nature of interpersonal family life for men by contributing an in-depth view of where, when and how they participate in family life. A major thesis of this book is that there is, and perhaps always has been, a disjuncture between the individualising accounts and representations of absent fathers and the complex, relational and dynamic character of the lived experiences of men themselves. The complex and often paradoxical relationship between the cultures and conduct of fathering is especially pertinent for men in low-income contexts, and perhaps more so than for fathers who are more resourced. In the contemporary context, it is only when we move away from spectacular accounts of absent fathers and deprived, fatherless communities that we are better able to develop a more sensitive comprehension of how low-income family life is 'done', organised, lived and sometimes contested from the perspectives of men whose relational and social ties and family experiences are all too often absented and rendered invisible. Narratives of the gendered and generational identities of men in low-income families both disrupt dominant discourses by contesting the pervasiveness of deficit thinking about men in low-income families, and invite acknowledgement of the fluid, relational and circumstantial nature of low-income family life. Substantially, MPLC offers a more complicated account of men's capabilities to engage in care across the lifecourse, albeit while negotiating precarity, (un)employment and family responsibilities in a context where state support continues to be withdrawn. The findings therefore develop the bigger picture, demonstrating how low-income family life creates opportunities for men to be more involved in caregiving, while also making it simultaneously challenging.

The dynamics of men's family lives: conceptualising family participation

Critical engagements with absent father discourses in the opening chapters of the book did not only prompt new research questions for exploring the perspectives of men experiencing family poverty, to sit alongside what we know about women and mothers. They were also central to the rationale for focused attention to how, when and why men participate in families, as well as when their participation might be constrained. To theorise the diverse experiences of low-income fathers and adult male carers in low-income contexts, the book therefore developed the conceptual language of family participation, as a new analytic lens that navigates the dynamics and complexities of low-income family life in the round. This conceptualisation moves beyond polarised framings of father absence and presence, aiming to address their limitations and to capture broader family change, including its patterns, responsibilities and interdependencies. Influenced and underscored by modes of fluid enquiry that are being advanced through QLR (Neale, 2019), the concept develops a dynamic and processual approach, influenced by an orientation to time and temporalities, which are beginning to have much greater influence in social and fathering research (Neale et al, 2015; Miller, 2018b). Attention to family participation enhances comprehension and explanation of diversity in men's care pathways, family roles, identities and generational responsibilities over time. It is therefore also likely to have application to an understanding of these processes and how they are experienced more generally.

The concept draws on and extends several interdisciplinary bodies of scholarship and an evidence base about involved fatherhoods that is predominantly empirically informed by the experiences of white, middle-class, heterosexual, married men (Dermott and Miller, 2015; Roy et al, 2015). The dominance of attention to fatherhood as a biological and ascribed identity also means that less is understood about diversity in caregiving by men across the lifecourse. This is especially problematic for developing an advanced understanding of low-income families. Indeed, family poverty scholars have identified that the experiences of fathers (and male carers) who are parenting in contexts of disadvantage constitute a key gap in contemporary knowledge (Ridge, 2009; Bennett and Daly, 2014). MPLC responded to acknowledgement of a paucity of evidence about how wider male family members, like uncles, brothers and grandfathers, participate in and sustain family lives; about the cumulative effect of living in conditions of poverty and disadvantage for men throughout the lifecourse; and about the influence of localities and communities on those experiences. Given that low-income families are more likely to express a range of dependencies on support services and men feel marginalised in support contexts because of their gender and a range of other intersecting social inequalities, qualitative evidence about their care responsibilities and family lives was sorely needed. The discussions and arguments of this book therefore foreground qualitative accounts by men themselves. Seeking to make visible the perspectives of men who are fathering 'from the margins' (Abdill, 2018; Elliott, 2020) in low-income families, this book has created a space to explore men's own views about their experiences of caring, how these arrangements came about, and what challenges they navigate and seek to overcome.

Family participation encapsulates men's varied pathways into care and the breadth of family and kinship practices, care arrangements and experiences that constitute their embeddedness in their family and community lives in low-income contexts. In this framing, family practices, or 'caring masculinities' (Elliott, 2016), that are enacted by men for and on behalf of families must be viewed in the context of an evolving and complex set of processes, experiences and obligations. The relational and interdependent nature of men's lives is emphasised, and a spectrum of responsibilities and practices in family contexts are encompassed that reflect the transitory nature of men's family responsibilities across the lifecourse. The study uncovered diverse forms of participation, from intensive caregiving where men have, or take up, primary paternal responsibilities including as lone parents, to limited involvements that reveal where, why and when there are limits to their participation. Also acknowledged are how longitudinal processes of deprivation and economic vulnerability are created, extended and/or sustained in ways that impact both on men's paternal responsibilities over time and on the wider sets of exchanges that are negotiated and contested within the long chains of gendered and intergenerational ties and relations that characterise family life.

Placed in the context of observations by professionals about the impacts of the practice and policy contexts that contoured the lives and experiences of men residing in the city (see Chapter 4), the empirical chapters of this book also presented three key dimensions that underscore this conceptualisation. Chapter 5 captured a diverse set of caring trajectories, arrangements and familial circumstances including young fathers whose claims to paternal responsibility were often undermined by a range of social disadvantages, lone, mid-life fathers with primary paternal responsibility and kinship carers. Chapter 6 identified the centrality of financial vulnerability to these processes and the provisioning practices required by men to manage them. These family practices and processes are also shaped by an increasingly punitive welfare offer and precarious and inflexible labour market. Chapter 7 revealed the limits to men's participation, demonstrating how men's identities can become disaggregated from family contexts, via processes of disconnection. In the context of the community centre or other locality-based resources, they seek alternative forms of belonging and citizenship in their localities and communities. In each of these chapters some consideration was given to the extent to which these men's diverse caring arrangements and familial generational positions were comparable, such that their circumstances either mitigated against, or intensified, the requirements for them to provide care in low-income families. While this varied hugely across the sample, there were also some common themes and conclusions that are drawn out further later in this chapter.

Significantly, the concept of family participation is better able to capture the diverse and crucial, yet often overlooked practices of care and support in which men engage in low-income family and community contexts. The MPLC data demonstrates fundamentally that families and family identities matter to men regardless of income and that men do engage in care and kinship, both in their everyday lives and across the lifecourse. It was evident that irrespective of generational position too, men embrace qualities of care and compassion, while also being responsive to needs and circumstances within families. As might be expected, given contemporary demographic trends and socioeconomic processes, the MPLC cases are reflective of complex patterns of family formation and practices of biological and social fathering. This includes child-rearing outside of marriage, across household and multiple-partner fertility, and multi-generational caregiving. Men's pathways into care were also wide ranging and driven by a combination of external circumstances and often constrained choice. Some of the young and lone fathers and male kinship carers actively sought to become primary caregivers for children, often in response to the needs of those children and through their visibility to a range of services and welfare agencies. Others were the only family members determined to be capable enough to take on care responsibilities for children. Their capability was determined either informally within families or formally, with external intervention.

Not only were there generational differences across the cases, but the family structures and relational circumstances of the men varied too. Some were lone fathers who had negotiated primary responsibility for children (in two cases, adult disabled children) with the mothers of their children and were committed to the long-term care of those children. Some gained primary responsibility for children in response to the needs and/or incapacity of the mothers of their children or other familial generations, usually because of a lack of financial resources. Of those who actively sought to gain primary responsibilities, most had negotiated complex legal processes to secure them.

Others were fathering while experiencing significant disadvantage themselves, linked to disability, economic vulnerability and age. These narratives sit alongside the more precarious care trajectories expressed by men accessing local resources and support whereby men had become increasingly isolated from family (for example, Chapter 7), offering both breadth and depth insights into men's caring responsibilities and trajectories over time. The concept of family participation therefore also benefits from an intersectional perspective that enriches knowledge of fathering and masculinities via considerations of diversity and inequalities. In capturing these diverse pathways, experiences and circumstances, the sample enabled comparison across the dataset of the diverging familial trajectories of men marginalised along various axes of social difference, namely their age, generation, (dis)ability, relationship status or residence in low-income families and/or localities.

An intersectional analysis of these data further demonstrates how some men in low-income contexts were able to individually disrupt gendered and classed assumptions and practices through their family participation and via the performance of caring masculinities (Elliott, 2016). While I developed some caution in Chapter 3 that caring masculinities may inadvertently be rendered ahistorical through their construction as being emergent in, and particular to, the contemporary moment, it is nonetheless a valuable concept for reintegrating men in family contexts and family interdependencies. It does so by explaining men's everyday investments in family support, provisioning and exchange, as well as their decision-making processes in relation to taking up or fulfilling their responsibilities towards children. From the perspective of poverty and family life, men's experiences were also brought to the fore to illustrate how, when and why men are present, revealing also where women are no longer able or available to support their families. In some instances, being a mum, a sister or expressing and fulfilling any other family identity is simply no longer enough to be able to provide care. In uncovering and exploring these diverse examples of fathering, enacted in a complex array of caring and familial arrangements, MPLC unveiled the gendered and intergenerational processes and obligations indicative of men's much wider familial involvement and intervention. These are not straightforwardly captured or explained through the languages of father involvement and absence.

Linked in part to the theoretical framework explained in Chapter 3, the concept has also been advanced to encapsulate the processes that shape men's lives as interdependent and linked across the lifecourse, regardless of socioeconomic status, age or gender. While men are often assumed to be at greater risk of social isolation and to lose functioning relationships in contexts of poverty and disadvantage (and Chapter 7 includes clear findings to confirm that these trajectories are a reality for some men), the men in this study had divergent trajectories that variably influenced a spectrum of family participation over time. Common to each of the participants was that they were always embedded in a complex web of interdependencies that were enacted both within and across households. Like Victor's narrative used in Chapter 1 to introduce the main themes of this book, it was evident that men are present in some relationships and disconnected from others. This finding has important implications for the methodologies and lenses that researchers employ to understand family lives, while also drawing attention to the social and relational dynamics of men's lifecourses and transitions and processes of deprivation. Additionally, men's relationships are almost always negotiated and contested across the lifecourse, worked out longitudinally and in the context of gendered and intergenerational relations with other family members.

Men's family participation was also determined in part by the changing welfare context of the UK. The partcipants' reflections on their social and relational lives were revealing of a wide range of intra- and intergenerational processes of caregiving, dependencies and material exchange that Conlon et al (2014: 140–141) suggest are characteristic of families with lower socioeconomic status in welfare contexts where investment in care is low:

> in lower socioeconomic groups, interdependencies between generations are more often reflected in the direct provision of care and support. The welfare state context matters because restricted availability of, and low public expenditure on, formal long-term care is one of the factors driving private expenditure on care by those who can afford it and recourse to family care for those who cannot.

As Brannen (2019) notes, family generational research presents mixed findings about whether families are safe havens in which resources are exchanged and members supported. Resource transfers within families are often contingent on family structure and solidarity, as well as on broader policy contexts including welfare regimes. As the most materially resourced prior to taking on care responsibilities unexpectedly, the older participants in MPLC demonstrated much greater choice and flexibility with regard to engaging in the rescue and repair (Emmel, 2017) of family ties and connections on behalf of their younger family members, even despite the hardships this produced. For the more marginalised and disadvantaged in the sample, including the young fathers and the single, mid-life fathers living in low-income localities, their social contexts meant that it was much harder to maintain such connections. In these cases, lack of resource is often interpreted as an individual problem and as men's lack of capability to provide care and maintain relationships. These comparisons demonstrate how men's connections to their familial lives and identities ebb and flow over time, shaped by dynamic processes of marginalisation and deprivation.

Even in situations where men had lost access to children or had become disconnected from their family contexts, they carried their familial identities and relationships forwards subjectively and sought to repair those connections or forge new social ties in their localities (for example, in neighbourhoods and communities, see Chapter 7). Investments in specific locality-based policy interventions are therefore a lifeline in such circumstances, supporting men to invest in new relationships, restore existing ones and establish a renewed sense of belonging. While susceptible to being viewed as the prototype for the selfish, irresponsible absent father who is depriving his children of a paternal figure, the complexities of these men's biographies and trajectories suggest that disconnection from families is influenced by marginalisation processes and inequalities rather than being simply a choice. This point is not made here to romanticise low-income men, to ignore their agency or even to claim representativeness. These findings were co-constructed between participants living in just one post-industrial city and a white, female researcher in a study whose lens was attuned to questions of men's family life and care. Nevertheless, they highlight the importance of refocusing attention on the contexts, structures and inequalities that shape the processes of men's family participation in low-income contexts. Here again, views of absence are largely debunked when rich, intimate movies of men's social worlds and experiences of low-income families and contexts are generated (Neale, 2019).

Overall, these findings lend weight to assertions that there is value in shifting the societal and academic focus away from how men in low-income families deprive their families and onto more dynamic, sociological questions about how and why particular contexts (familial, practice, policy, localities and so on) might deprive men of their family lives or produce occasions that require more intensive involvement yet impinge on their capabilities to sustain their family participation. This not only includes depriving them of opportunities for family participation and the forms of engagement that they may desire, but also depriving them of visibility and recognition for the valuable contributions that they do make. These deprivations of context, as processes that marginalise men from family contexts, are considered in the next section.

The deprivations of context

While the previous section developed a case for foregrounding and conceptualising men's family participation by bringing men's roles and responsibilities back into visibility and analysing the experiences of men as active participants in family life, another key argument is that the contexts in which these men are supporting and sustaining their families are increasingly challenging and often mitigate against their efforts, producing considerable barriers and constraints. The study therefore advances analyses of the contexts of significant hardship through which men in low-income family and community contexts engage in a range of caring practices. These analyses showcase new narratives of caring masculinities as they play out through a broader historical and policy context of austerity that is entrenching conditions antithetical to these men's efforts on behalf of their children, grandchildren and wider family members. While the notion of 'dad deprivation' (Ashe, 2014) invoked in policy and public arenas infers a lack or absence of men from households as fathers, especially from the lives of boys and young men, the study findings provide impetus and rationale for a radical reclaiming of the concept. They do so through an examination of the contexts and processes through which men become increasingly materially deprived when invested in family life and are, themselves, dads deprived. Longitudinal analyses comparing men in different generational positions reveal both circumstances where men might be more resourced and capable of taking on care responsibilities, and also circumstances where state and/or labour market support is lacking yet much needed.

As the opening quotes of this book by young father Tommy (FYF) and grandfather Victor (IGE) demonstrate, men are present in low-income family contexts and express a distinct desire to be there for their children. Across the entire corpus of data from the three studies, there was evidence that the older men were much more able to demonstrate and fulfil these expectations, either in their commitments as primary caregivers to their children and/or in their engagements with external agencies on behalf of their children (including the courts and child protection processes). In these ways, their intentions and desires around their responsibilities and family relationships are no different than those expressed by involved fathers and might be conceived as evidence of what Elliott (2020) conceptualises as transformative caring masculinities emerging among marginalised men (in this study low-income fathers). Roberts and Elliott (2020) are critical of the notion that problematic masculinities are typically considered the preserve of marginalised men and importantly trouble the idea that privileged men are best positioned to drive transformation and progress in masculinities. MPLC lends further empirical weight to this argument with its focus on low-income fathers and their family participation. While engaging with universal expectations and discourses of involved and good fatherhood, the family practices and caring arrangements of these participants were evidence of how this was achieved via their intensive support for children. However, the consequences for men when they are unable to do this can be pernicious, leading to trajectories of disconnection and isolation.

Despite overlaps with middle-class and resourced men in terms of expressed and, in most cases, realised intentions to 'be there', this study has revealed how the contexts around these men's experiences produce unique hardships. The roles and responsibilities of the MPLC study were occurring in contexts where the men's ability to balance their earning capacities with family care were perhaps most subject to compromise or challenge. As noted, cutting across the different generational categories of the participant group, the fathers in this study were diverse in terms of their partnership status, situation in the lifecourse, generational position, history of fathering and (dis)ability or impairment experience, but all were in situations that render families financially vulnerable.

They also described a range of parenting categories that are often problematised (for example, Kilkey and Clarke, 2010) or rendered invisible. Some were lone fathers; some were non-resident; some were parenting with a disability or parenting a disabled adult child; some were stigmatised because of their age and generational position; and some were unemployed or socially excluded. These categorisations were subject to change over time and, in most cases, were contoured by much longer intergenerational histories of deprivation and neglect. Men's family participation must therefore be acknowledged as an outcome of much longer family histories and of the intergenerational and relational processes and exchanges that are inherent to family contexts. These have ripple effects both within and across family contexts and over time. To talk simply about involved and/or absent fathers is to decouple men from their personal and familial relations and to decontextualise their experiences and the ways in which they become responsible for a child. It is pertinent to note here also that in the current economic and political climate of austerity, which represents the most advanced neoliberal policy state for many years, the range of family, employment, welfare and youth policies that impact on families has become increasingly punitive.

In longitudinal and intergenerational perspective, a notable paradox identified here, then, is that low-income family life creates opportunities for men to be more involved in caregiving, while also making it simultaneously challenging. However, the nature of these challenges varied for each generational cohort. While perhaps most resourced and able to take on care responsibilities for children, the older men often did so unexpectedly. These participants therefore described the weight of the decisions they had to make about taking on often unanticipated care responsibilities, in some cases engaging in complex and what they described as gender-biased processes through the courts and in engagements with professionals that are difficult to negotiate. These decisions are not just about whether providing care is the right thing to do. While primary care responsibilities for children can be emotionally rewarding and fulfilling, they can also come at significant financial, material and emotional cost. Many of these participants were, and became, financially vulnerable themselves and were experiencing economic hardship. They therefore demonstrated their capability for providing stable environments for children, but in many cases did so in constrained financial circumstances.

To some extent, the older men were more financially protected than the younger men in the sample, especially if they had histories of secure employment and savings. However, these were quickly diminished, particularly where care was required for multiple children. The case of kinship carer Theo, introduced in Chapter 6, is relevant in this regard. Having depleted his life savings and those of his mother so as to keep his nieces and nephews together, he was left with no more than £3.26 a day to support them while state support was being negotiated. Cases like Theo's indicate not that men deprive their children or younger family members but that contemporary societal caring arrangements are such that grandparents and family members who take on care responsibilities become quickly deprived by societal and welfare contexts. Poor financial provisioning for care and unpaid labour make it increasingly difficult for them to provide for their families. A toxic constellation of deprivations like these may also have catastrophic impacts for young people. For example, when the most resourced family members become deprived too, when men are not acknowledged as possible carers and their lives are made increasingly precarious through poor financial resourcing and inaccessible, inflexible work, there is a much greater risk that children will be removed from family contexts altogether.

Interrogating the contexts of opportunity and constraint that men manage and navigate in order to make decisions about their families and how they sustain them further challenges existing explanatory frameworks about how family processes and practices either reproduce or unsettle existing hierarchies and inequalities. For these participants, the wider variety of alternative ways of living that they express is *not necessarily what they choose* because they are on low income, but because these are *the only options that are left to them* because they have a low income. As a theoretical contribution, these findings demonstrate that, in contexts of marginalised fatherhoods, the doing of kinship and the fulfilment of kin responsibilities often also supersedes the gender of the person. The question here is not whether men are or are not caring but rather that being a dad, a grandad, an uncle, a brother and so on are important identities for these men and strongly influence their decisions to maintain and strengthen their connections with their children or even to take on unforeseen care responsibilities later in life. Thus, generational identities, which have an inherently relational character, are a key explanatory factor in how and why men engage in family participation both later in the lifecourse and despite the poverty and hardship that may create or exacerbate. These findings lend weight to arguments by Featherstone et al (2017) that family poverty itself should be upheld as a form of societal neglect rather than the individual responsibility of adult family members.

However, this is not to say that gender is not an important explanatory factor in these processes. The participants described processes that were gendered in a variety of ways and that impacted on their lived experiences and biographies in ways that reflected those that might be expected because they were men. The young fathers interviewed aspired to the package deal identified by Townsend (2002) and expressed the conventional aspirations of a male lifecourse: a family, a home and stable employment. However, the limitations of their contexts meant that they often became disconnected from families and from the labour market and sought belonging in their communities and localities instead. Sam, as a kinship carer, compared his role as caregiver more favourably to the situations of men of a similar age, whom he perceived as withering away in working-men's clubs. In these cases, men aren't straightforwardly marginalised from family life in the ways that are implied and encompassed in the policy framing of absence (which really refers to absence by choice both from the household and economic provisioning), although gendered expectations and ideologies remain relevant to how they interpret their experiences.

Observations of the longitudinal dynamics of deprivation made possible through analytic attention to men's familial and generational identities are also revealing of the gendered and classed processes and trajectories that either require men to step in to sustain family life (typically for their younger family members in the case of the older participants) or serve to disconnect men from their families altogether. Compared with the trajectories and caring arrangements of the older men, the cases of the young fathers and those living in low-income localities (for example, Chapter 7) are illustrative of how boys and men appear to be at greater risk of becoming disconnected from families and isolated much earlier in the lifecourse than women. McDowell (2014) theorises this as linked in part to the change in sexual contract between mothers and their teenage sons, but local context and community also play a key role here. The MPLC findings offer additional evidence that young men's trajectories of connection and interdependence as they transition to adulthood are risk laden and have become increasingly precarious. Increasingly, perilous access to the labour market, and the sociability that secure connections to employment engender, have been eroded, and when young fathers do find employment the exploitative, unrewarding and degrading nature of the work impinges on their family life both financially and in terms of time. In low-income localities, the alternative trajectories or 'biographical careers' (MacDonald and Shildrick, 2007) available to young men can be exclusionary and marked by unpredictability. Creating their own families can be a protective factor, but the stakes are high in a welfare and policy context where policy support for men has lagged, welfare has been stripped to the bone and is fragmented and men's engagements in caring continue to be considered suspect or problematic.

From a comparative perspective, these processes also had differential effects on the men, dependent on their age and generational positions, highlighting the essential role of employing an intersectional lens that is attentive to inequalities of age and generation, as well as gender and class. Men's capacities for family participation are contoured by wider structural processes and are either enabled or constrained by the material and social resources available to them. Employment, household finances, housing, availability of formal and informal supports in localities and the extent of the need of their child(ren) variously shaped men's decision making and abilities to do the right thing by their families. Accessing employment was especially problematic for the young men in the sample, who described dissatisfaction with the exploitative, door-to-door work available. In many instances it did not pay, was unrewarding and impinged on important time that could be spent with children. Where labour market opportunities were available, the hours were often inflexible and organisations did not see men as carers and thus would not accommodate childcare requirements. These findings support existing evidence that men especially struggle to find part-time and flexible work in the current economy because traditional gender norms and ideologies around parenthood continue to operate in organisations (Yeandle et al, 2003; Gatrell et al, 2015). The requirements and increasingly punitive conditionality of welfare support also clash with men's ability to balance childcare with finding work, and the older men in the sample interpreted this as a kind of 'labour' being forced for the purposes of a tick-box exercise. For those at the sharp end of hardship, including those whom I met at the community centre, the requirements to catch multiple buses in order to sign on at the Job Centre not only increased their hardships but had little to no effect on the structural inequalities they were already experiencing.

The precarity of youth transitions in the austerity context has also increased and the uneven effects on already disadvantaged populations have been exacerbated. Young men in the most deprived circumstances are coming to the age of work at a time where employment opportunities are increasingly scarce and the only work available is low paid and insecure. Young men must either present themselves as work-ready neoliberal subjects, as 'individualised entrepreneurs', or, regardless of their existing dependents, care responsibilities or residence in towns where work for the less-skilled has all but vanished, become labelled as shirkers (McDowell, 2017). The reduction in welfare entitlements linked to austerity (Neale and Davies, 2015a), has further deepened these inequalities, shaping and intensifying young men's experiences of exclusion and marginalisation and the forging of ever more diverse and precarious trajectories to adulthood (Gunter and Watt, 2009). Austerity policies have increased the vulnerabilities of young, working-class men and boys who, for the first time in several generations, have worse prospects for social mobility than their parents (McDowell, 2017). This study has demonstrated the erosive and isolating effect this can have on young men seeking to establish and provide for their own families, and the essential role of welfare and support services in working with young fathers to fulfil their ambitions to be involved as fathers while also managing their employment fortunes.

Despite typically having more of a financial buffer than the young men, many of the older men in this study were also struggling to re-enter the workforce in their late 50s and early 60s and felt awkwardly positioned by the state with regard to financial recompense. This was specifically raised by the kinship carers who reported being asked by social services to leave employment in order to settle their children and were then later being asked how they intended to support those children financially in the longer term. A lack of transparency and clarity about welfare entitlements could additionally result in significant debt and stress. Especially challenging for the fathers who were responsible for school-age children is finding paid work that is flexible enough to accommodate school holidays and hours. The soaring costs of childcare for younger children and lack of flexibility also mean that work often does not pay. This is even harder in deprived contexts where employment is low wage and long hours. The combination of meeting the unrealistic expectations of welfare conditionality to seek and hold down insecure or inappropriate work alongside the ongoing and inherently sexist and ageist nature of organisational cultures also works together to mitigate against men's capabilities to care, both assumed and realised.

Supporting men as fathers and carers

What might these findings mean for policy and practice? Families have long been considered carers by default, especially when normative imperatives align with the structural absence of formal support and options (Keating et al, 2019). Given the recency of the COVID-19 pandemic and the likelihood of other serious socioeconomic transformation in future linked to Brexit, the COVID-19 pandemic and other, as yet unknowable, events, there is a need to think seriously about how policy makers offer meaningful protection for families and support them to improve their capacity to manage the wider shocks and forces that produce family instability.

In line with recent research literatures about the impacts of austerity and welfare reforms on families (for example, Jupp, 2017; Greer Murphy, 2019; Hall, 2019), MPLC sought to demonstrate the significance for policy making of considering the everyday lived experiences and narratives of families as lived from below. The outcomes and findings of MPLC, including those generated with professionals and elaborated in Chapter 4, are most likely to be of relevance to national policy makers and local agencies and services that provide family support or that engage with fathers or adult male carers. It is evident that men with primary caring responsibilities in low-income families remain highly isolated, so it is important that compassionate support is available that recognises why and when men are vulnerable and that champions their participation in family life.

There is compelling evidence to suggest that mainstream welfare and market provision plays a role in contributing to men's isolation and marginalisation, meaning that support for their family participation is neither being produced nor sustained. From a policy perspective, UK family policies ostensibly promote father involvement and discourage absence. However, the nature and character of father absence is little understood and, as this book illustrates, is more complex and dynamic than is often acknowledged. There is evident need for greater attention to the ways in which welfare and labour market conditions can be developed so that they impact in more positive and progressive ways on family lives and enable men's participation to flourish, rather than punish and mitigate against their efforts. A key premise for much research and policy that champions the value of involved fathers is that when men are positively engaged in family life there are widespread individual, familial and societal benefits. More broadly, there is persuasive evidence to suggest that men's involvement in family contexts can alleviate gendered inequalities and that their participation is an important mechanism in progress towards gender equality (Boyer et al, 2017; van der Gaag et al, 2019; Brooks and Hodkinson, 2020). However, progress in this direction is often hampered by structural inequalities and social discourses that discredit and demonise men and are still found in the approaches of professionals. The findings here suggest an issue at the heart of progress in this direction, highlighting how current welfare and labour market processes may inadvertently discriminate against and exclude those who do not have the resources available to achieve gender equality.

In the Slovenian context, Hrženjak (2017) finds that the intensification, flexibilisation and precaritisation characteristic of the contemporary labour market and the near-permanent state of economic crisis that is being sustained by austerity policies are having the effect of eroding men's rights as workers (and caregivers), producing uncertainty and limiting their autonomy with regard to family participation. Hrženjak's research identifies how gender relations are more likely to be retraditionalised among parents in couples where labour market attachments are insecure and precarious. Advancing these findings, MPLC, which interviewed men in different generational positions and family circumstances who were variously 'deprivileged marginalised groups in the labour market' (Hrženjak, 2017), shows how current welfare and labour market processes undermine men's efforts in already non-traditional family and gendered circumstances. This research therefore suggests that much greater attention needs to be given at policy level to the economic and structural factors that facilitate men (and women) to resist gendered work and care norms across a much wider spectrum of family configurations. Furthermore, support for these diverse forms of family participation and caring arrangements is essential, especially when they involve keeping families together. This kind of work will involve investment, a cohesive national policy strategy that gives attention to men as caregivers and a range of stakeholder groups and organisations who recognise and nurture men's capabilities regardless of their familial identity. At the level of family policy, there is also more work to be done to promote an improved and greater range of entitlements that enable the sustainable uptake of care by men, especially alongside employment (see Boyer et al, 2017). Change in organisational cultures that enable men to request more flexible, part-time working is an essential piece of this complex policy landscape.

Men in low-income contexts are also likely to have some dependency on local support services at some point in their caring trajectories, and in some cases at least some involvement with statutory agencies. As evidenced here and in wider literatures, low-income families are more likely to engage locally because they are both materially and financially restricted (MacDonald et al, 2005; Daly and Kelly, 2015), highlighting the significant role of place-based services in supporting these men in their efforts on behalf of their families. However, the great deal of care, support and nurturing provided by men in low-income families often remains unknown to service providers and hidden from view. When men do come into view, they often report encounters with systems and professionals that subject them to surveillance or construct them as a risk. Such practices reflect gender bias in service approaches and are underpinned by a risk ethos, rather than one of redemption and resource (Ladlow and Neale, 2016). There are convincing emerging arguments that, regardless of generational position, men value support that is premised on an ethos of care and commitment (Neale and Davies, 2015b; Ward et al, 2017; Tarrant and Neale, 2017a).

The study findings render these important forms of family participation more visible, while also promoting new knowledge and understanding of the complex range of issues faced both by men with primary care responsibilities in low-income families and by those who reside in low-income contexts and may be at heightened risk of isolation. This research therefore offers new insights about some of the complexities that policy makers and practitioners might be faced with in their intentions to support capacity building within families so that they can prosper. Consequently, effective policy and practice for men is required that is also responsive to lifecourse dynamics and diversity in their experiences (Tarrant and Neale, 2017a). The concept of family participation may be useful here, rather than the idea of father involvement, which tends to reify time spent with children rather than the quality of emotional connection and strength of familial and kinship identities that influence men's decisions (constrained as they may be) to take up parental responsibilities over the lifecourse. The men who participated in this research were engaged in essential roles to foster the well-being and resilience of their families, demonstrating that they were inherently capable of providing safe family environments even in contexts of hardship. In some cases, they were choosing to do so often in challenging and unanticipated circumstances that were impoverishing in and of themselves. When we recognise that men make decisions about their family lives relationally, that is, not just as men but because they have a range of generational and familial identities, as fathers, grandfathers, uncles, brothers, nephews and so on, then we may be better able to support them in their efforts towards their families.

Returning to an earlier point, I would also concur with a developing argument for a radical reframing of support where men's fathering and caring roles, and men themselves, are acknowledged as a resource, rather than a risk to their families. The pervasive framework of risk is wide reaching and confirmed by the MPLC findings and there is compelling wider evidence to suggest that, regardless of age, socioeconomic, generational position, race and so on, fathers and wider male family members remain on the periphery of service delivery (Neale and

Davies, 2015b; Brandon et al, 2017; Tarrant and Neale, 2017a, 2017b, also see Chapter 4). They are not always seen as the 'core business' of support (Zanoni et al, 2013), especially if they are not biologically related. Where men put themselves forward to services as potential carers they are not always given the time or support they need. Barriers therefore remain in relationships between male family members and practitioners such that they are not always recognised or supported as possible caregivers. These barriers may be reinforced via gendered thinking in working relationships (Philip et al, 2018), as evidenced by the subtle judgements the men in MPLC described, such as having a 'manly' or unfurnished house (for example, Sam and Shaun, also see Philip et al, 2018). When wider cultural ideas around gendered roles and identities in low-income contexts become an impediment, the stakes are high. There are cases here where men were overlooked as potential carers or were given limited time and opportunity to put themselves forward (for example, Shane's case). There is therefore a need for a gender-sensitive response that acknowledges how processes of caregiving, especially those that require some form of formal intervention, are gendering, may inadvertently reinforce inequalities and limit recognition of men's care.

For children who encounter the child protection system the stakes are even higher, especially where men are regarded as risks. In feeding back insights from the male kinship carers who participated in the study to the national charity Grandparents Plus (rebranded Kinship in March 2021) toward the end of the study, it was observed that when men are not considered as potential carers or supported to be when they choose to become primary caregivers, the risk is that children will be removed from family contexts altogether. In their reflections on research with low-income mid-life grandparents, Hughes and Emmel (2011) suggest that policy and practice provision should widen their scope to recognise the vital roles grandparents (and wider family members like brothers, uncles and so on) play in giving their grandchildren a good start in life. This should include grandfathers and wider adult male family members too. MPLC demonstrates the need to recognise the essential roles that may be enacted by a diverse range of family members regardless of their gender, age, generation and other differences. While the council employees whose narratives were discussed in Chapter 4 reflect an awareness of the significance of seeing children as relational actors who are embedded in family contexts with varying degrees of resource, the tendency to lapse into now debunked theories of intergenerational cycles of deprivation and absent fatherhood precluded the contributions of those men who could provide care and support beyond the parent generation. Agencies and professionals who think critically and reflexively about the policy assumptions that individualise low-income families, by recognising how wider socioeconomic contexts and structural constraints might mitigate against men's efforts to participate in and sustain family life, are currently better placed to provide the tailored and flexible support that is often required.

Men are also especially likely to need support and guidance when there is some form of legal intervention that impinges on ostensibly private familial contexts. This is true for separated families when child maintenance issues arise and in cases where there is an imposition of rules on the family on the grounds of gender difference, men are at particular risk of accusations of sexual misconduct, representing a major source of relational stress and tension within families. In both cases, they (and their partners) need support to understand and manage requirements. Furthermore, in the context of kinship care arrangements there are at least two cases in this small sample of 26 where boys had been separated from female siblings. Such rules are linked to the provision of adequate space via social housing, but they are also made on a distinction of gender difference, rather than family ties and relationships. For young boys who have lost parents to premature death or because of neglect, this is especially problematic. Maintaining family connectedness would potentially have represented a 'safer' option in the ostensibly extreme but remarkably similar cases of the grandson of kinship carer Paul and of Ashley, for example, who demonstrate trajectories of separation from the family, placement in a children's home, collective engagements with other boys that are comparable to gangs, and then trajectories characterised by criminal justice involvement.

It is also important to re-emphasise that while the men in this study were holding their families together, they were doing so in a context where the resources they had at their disposal were limited or steadily declining. In the decade since 2010, political austerity has exacerbated the conditions in which men are more likely to be required to take on care responsibilities. Yet they are also required to do so in a welfare environment that is increasingly punitive in its emphasis on securing work and placing limits on financial resources both within and across households and within different sets of interdependencies to incentivise employment. These challenges are likely to be compounded further in the post-Brexit and COVID-19 pandemic environments of the UK. Both are already having profound and disproportionate socioeconomic impacts, in ways that we can anticipate will produce new ruptures in social and cultural experience while simultaneously reinforcing existing inequalities. However, as Boyer et al (2017) note, while recessionary (and related political) processes can have negative effects, they may also present opportunities for more progressive work/care arrangements and gender-equitable divisions of labour. Crucially, though, in agreement with a compelling argument made by Bonner-Thomson and McDowell (2020), uncovering and rendering these men's practices of caregiving more visible in these contexts should not be simply read as a form of resilience in these men and their families that absolves the state and right-wing governments of any responsibility. The findings, supported by other research evidence and practice developments, demonstrate a need to develop more father-inclusive but gender-sensitive practice, policy and organisational environments that are of benefit to anyone with care responsibilities (Tarrant and Neale, 2017a, 2017b).

This study has demonstrated that investments in compassionate and progressive family support, especially in deprived localities, can enable men to repair relationships and connections in their own lives through either the facilitation of renewed forms of belonging or the repair of processes that affect and disadvantage younger family members. There is also a clear and continued role here for policy makers and practitioners to promote the value of men's participation in low-income family contexts (also see Henwood et al, 2010), regardless of their generational position in the family and familial circumstances, and to seek to support them to remove constraints to their participation. More generally, this requires professionals and policy makers to see men as family members and not just as gendered subjects. There is also potential that a lack of familial resources and disadvantage will become conflated with lack of capability, as is often the case with young fathers (Neale et al, 2015). This requires policy makers and professionals to listen with empathy and to acknowledge what impinges on men's efforts towards their families and deprives them in such circumstances. Such an approach should also help to reduce burdens on families when the state intervenes.

These arguments only bolster evidence of the necessity to critique ideas of intergenerational poverty, worklessness and father absence, the 'zombie arguments' (MacDonald et al, 2014) that have been subject to frequent sociological critique yet continually experience a resurgence, dominate policy agendas and scapegoat individual fathers and their families. As suggested by the professionals who adopted more compassionate and context-aware approaches to the circumstances of the men they engaged with, there is a need instead to consider how public and third sector services, relationships and policy interventions might operate in more inclusive ways with men with care responsibilities and who are experiencing long-term poverty in ways that their voices and perspectives directly inform and promote positive changes. A key question here is *how* this might be achieved and what processes drive such change. These mechanisms for change are being considered in my current and ongoing research that builds directly out of the collaborations and connections established in the MPLC study. In the final section of this chapter, I highlight my own ongoing research and future opportunities and priorities in a post-Brexit and COVID-19 pandemic context.

Ongoing and future research

While this book goes some way towards challenging the idea that men in low-income families are an area of empirical neglect, by synthesising existing evidence sources in the literature and uncovering more recent data histories via qualitative secondary analysis, there is scope to strengthen the evidence base further.

Building directly out of the MPLC study, I am now taking forward an ambitious new agenda in research and engagement with young fathers (aged 25 and under). With £1.2 million of funding under the UK Research and Innovation Future Leaders Fellowship scheme, Following Young Fathers Further (FYFF) commenced in January 2020 and aims to extend knowledge of the parenting journeys and support needs of young fathers. This four-year study is employing qualitative longitudinal, participatory and comparative methods to advance the existing evidence base, developing both extended and international comparative evidence.

In the current UK welfare and policy context, young parents are often constructed as a risk and a problem (Duncan, 2010). Young fathers are more likely than any other age group of fathers to bear the brunt of stigmatising, classist and, indeed, ageist assumptions that underpin wider policy concerns about absent fatherhood. Recent contributions to the literature on young parenthood highlight how young fathers can be positively involved in family life when given effective familial and service support across their parenting journeys (Neale et al, 2015; Tarrant and Neale, 2017a, b). However, young men continue to carve out their fathering identities in a structural context where stereotypes of dead-beat and feckless young dads are rampant. Young fathers particularly face a range of socioeconomic inequalities and adverse life experiences that can make positive involvement in their children's lives more challenging. Thus, despite compelling evidence that they desire to be engaged in their children's lives, they continue to experience exclusion and stigmatisation, including in professional support contexts (Tarrant and Neale, 2017b). There is therefore a pressing need to see young fathers in a different way and to turn these common-sense, yet often unfounded, ideas on their head.

FYFF is a significant and exciting opportunity to both implement and document a compassionate and participatory social policy and support environment in the UK by generating a longitudinal evidence base and implementing practice solutions co-created with young fathers, family and other support services that are of benefit for young fathers, their families and wider civil society. There is also enormous potential for methodological innovation, enabling advances in qualitative secondary analysis and extended qualitative longitudinal and comparative work with cohorts of young fathers and with professionals who can inform policy and practice.

Of course, the COVID-19 pandemic that has resulted in extended periods of government intervention and lockdown policies enforcing social distancing in countries across the world, that were first imposed in March 2020 in the UK, is the biggest global social crisis of a generation. Emerging social-scientific evidence already indicates that the lockdowns, as recurrent public health interventions, are having disproportionate impacts for low-income families and are exacerbating existing inequalities. While it is tempting to frame the pandemic as an isolated and 'unprecedented' moment, social scientists are well placed to raise awareness of and to provide explanations for the differential impacts of the pandemic as it unfolds, including on personal and family arrangements and everyday life. In its first wave of interviews the FYFF study has examined the impacts of the unfolding crisis on young fathers and their support needs (Tarrant et al, 2020a, 2020b). It has become imperative for social scientists, now more than ever, to research through this crisis and to advise on policy and practice as it emerges to deal with the social impacts of the pandemic. Social-historical evidence also has a significant place in this.

APPENDIX A

Participant information

Table A.1: Core 'Men, Poverty and Lifetimes of Care' participants

Pseudonym	Age	Employment status	Care status	Method
Adrian	18	Unemployed	Non-resident father	Life journey interview
Andrew	70	Unemployed	Grandfather/stepfather	Life journey interview
Andy	30	Unemployed	Non-resident father	Life journey interview
Ashley	22	Charity fundraiser	Stepfather	Life journey interview Photovoice
Connor	16	In college	Non-resident father	Life journey interview
Damien	14	In school	Secondary carer (father)	Life journey interview
Dean	26	Unemployed	Secondary carer (father)	Life journey interview
Dougie	73	Retired	Kinship carer	Life journey interview
Earle	72	Retired	Grandfather	Life journey interview
Graham	45	Unemployed	Non-resident father	Life journey interview Walking photovoice
Joe	22	Unemployed	Non-resident father	Life journey interview
Joseph	45	Unemployed	Lone father	Life journey interview Photovoice
Lewis	38	Unemployed	Stepfather	Life journey interview
Marvin	61	Unemployed	Grandfather	Life journey interview
Matthew	55	Unemployed	Lone father	Life journey interview Photovoice
Paul	52	Retired	Kinship carer	Life journey interview
Pearce	57	Unemployed	Kinship carer	Life journey interview
Reece	22	Employed	Secondary carer (father)	Life journey interview
Reggie	55	Unemployed	Kinship carer	Life journey interview Photovoice

(continued)

Table A.1: Core 'Men, Poverty and Lifetimes of Care' participants (continued)

Pseudonym	Age	Employment status	Care status	Method
Ricky	22	Unemployed	Lone father	Life journey interview
Rory	61	Unemployed	Lone father	Life journey interview
Sam	51	Unemployed	Kinship carer	Life journey interview
Shane	27	Unemployed	Kinship carer	Life journey interview
Shaun	38	Unemployed	Lone father	Life journey interview
Theo	38	Unemployed	Kinship carer	Life journey interview
Will	44	Unemployed	Non-resident father	Life journey interview Walking photovoice

Other members of the community centre took part in the walking photovoice, including Jed and Bill, young mum Jodie and her friend Leanne (see Chapter 7). Given the nature of the methods used, demographic data was not generated for these participants.

'Existing evidence' document shared at the knowledge-exchange workshop

The following text has been reproduced from a pamphlet called 'Existing Evidence' that I shared at the knowledge-exchange workshop discussed in Chapter 4.

Men, Poverty and Lifetimes of Care

While a growing body of qualitative research is beginning to emerge about the 'lived experiences' of low-income families living in poverty, the experiences of family men (that is, fathers and grandfathers) and the cumulative effects of living in conditions of poverty and disadvantage are still significant gaps in knowledge.

In response, two sets of archived qualitative longitudinal data, held in a research archive at the University of Leeds (Timescapes), have been analysed: (1) to explore men's everyday and long-term experiences of family life when living on a low-income and (2) to generate new research questions that derive from, and take into account, these findings. The first dataset, Following Young Fathers (FYF), provides evidence of the experiences of teenage fathers; the second, IGE, contains narratives of the lived experiences of mid-life grandparents (including grandfathers). Both sets of participants live in low-income localities in a northern city in England, and the datasets when brought together show the diverse ways in which men experience poverty and social exclusion over time, influencing the extent of support and care that they can provide and that they also receive.

In this pamphlet I present fragments of the stories of the men from both datasets to demonstrate that men value their roles as fathers and grandfathers but that, over time, they struggle to balance their responsibilities within particularly constrained circumstances. My intention is that these findings resonate with you and your own practice, and it would be really beneficial to explore those questions that you think will best support you, both in your practice and in policy making. All of the quotations used in this pamphlet are from the participants that were interviewed for the two archived projects and have been anonymised.

Men are committed to the people in their families and value their roles as fathers and grandfathers

Across the datasets, men engage in a range of care practices. Most of the men are fathers and grandfathers and they value these roles highly. They describe parenting as a process, and one that is learnt over time. For young men, fathering is a positive and valued role. Aspirations for fatherhood provide them with motivation and emancipate them from the trappings of their localities. For older men, grandfatherhood is a second chance to parent again and to learn from mistakes made in the past:

'It's changed my personality and who I am and that. I mean I used to be a right little ... but yeah I've, it's made me realise that I need to do good and that and try and stay out of trouble and, so yeah ... I mean if I didn't have them I wouldn't have, I probably wouldn't be like this. I won't, well I know I would have gone into college and done all that. But it's made me stronger. It's made me look towards my life and yeah so it's changed me a lot yeah ... yeah motivated. It's just put me in right direction. It's made me think "oh look I've, I've gotta show 'em that, how to be a good dad when they are older". And you need to bring them up right and that. And that's how I've seen it, so yeah.' (Callum, age 19, father of twins, separated (FYF))

'Well, I always say that having grandkids gives you a second chance at life, you know what I mean cos you've learnt by your mistakes ... and now you can only teach them, you know what I mean. Cos when you first get married, you get kids, hey there is no manual you know, saying do this do that. You've got to learn by your mistakes, haven't you?' Interviewer: Yeah, yeah. 'But I mean once you've learnt that and you've got your grandkids, you've realised then that you know what to do.' (Bob, age 56, grandfather (IE))

As well as being fathers and grandfathers, men also look out for each other in their localities as uncles and brothers

> 'Like I'm not close wi' ma mum at all. We always fight. I'm close wi' ma grandma but not as close as what I am wi' ma two uncles. It's like one a' ma uncles, he's always looked after me. And like if anyone's hurt me he's always gone and stuck up for me. And ma other uncle, he's like, he's always there for me to talk to. And he's helped me with money and that. Like if I need money, he'll give me it.' (Jimmy, age 16 (FYF))

Interviewer:	You stopped [younger brother] doing what you and [Jamie's twin brother] had done [getting in trouble around the estate].
Jamie (son of Sheila (IE)):	Well that's obvious, he's my younger brother, you know what I mean, I wouldn't let him do the things what I did when I was younger, I might not have been caught for anything like it, you know what I mean, but it still, I didn't do it, but I still want, I wouldn't want my younger brother to do it.

However, over time, men may be unable to fulfil their care responsibilities because of continuing constraints on their resources

For a variety of reasons, including ongoing constraints on their time, money and relationships, men's choices can become harder and they are not always supported in the fulfilment of their caring responsibilities. Some examples of this are outlined here.

Geography, relationships with partners and a lack of state support

The young men want to be involved in their children's lives but face a number of constraints. Living on a low income makes it difficult to see children, especially if fathers are non-resident, like Jake, and if ex-partners and their families are controlling access. In the long term, legal processes are costly and Legal Aid is harder to access, rendering some men additionally vulnerable in terms of being able to fulfil their care responsibilities.

> 'I can't go up there every day and she can't, well she don't wanna come to mine. And like I want to see Riley. So if she don't want to bring him to see me or she won't let me take him out then it'd have to go through courts wouldn't it. And I don't wanna do that cos then it'll just cause bigger, worse argument.' (Jimmy, age 17, non-resident, in a volatile relationship (FYF))

Interviewer:	If legal aid was still that in place do you think you would have contacted the solicitors?
Richard (age 16, separated (FYF)):	Yeah, straight away. She knows that I'm getting cash in hand so she can't like do anything,
Interviewer:	What do you mean she can't do anything?
Richard:	She like, she's been saying like, "oh I'm taking you to CSA". I said, "go on then".
Interviewer:	Oh, right.
Richard:	And stuff like this. I said, "listen you aren't getting no money off me. If she [daughter] wants stuff, tell me what she wants and I'll go get it myself so I know you're not wasting money on this, that and the other. So I know that I'm buying it, the money's going on her, not you." Do you know what I mean?

Men are not just 'absent' dads. They make decisions about their responsibilities in relation to their resources and within complex family circumstances

The issue of child maintenance is complex and, at present, does not support men to fulfil their care responsibilities across the lifecourse. Daniel would prefer to care for his son full time rather than pay child maintenance to his ex-partner. Victor has multiple care responsibilities and is highly invested in the lives of his step-children, foster children and step-grandchild in his current marriage. However, several factors mean that he is viewed as an absent father by the Child Support Agency. In both examples, men's lives remain tied to the circumstances of their ex-partners.

'At the moment she hasn't approached me for maintenance, which I feel … once she either goes into full-time work or if she goes … to university or whatever … I think she's going to approach me. I can't imagine why she wouldn't approach me. It seems to be in her favour to get money outta me. Which is very annoying when I've been forced into this predicament and on top of it, I'm being told "you're paying this money". It's like "well I'll have him full time" [laughs].' (Dominic, age 19, separated, works full time (FYF))

'From when I left my ex, I was paying her maintenance, but she was refusing to let me see [son from previous relationship] … my ex-partner, she's never worked and she's always sat on benefits, which then affected what happened to me, then, with the Child Support Agency … What she did was, she took two part-time jobs, the emphasis then was on me … They weren't legal jobs. The emphasis was then on me to grass her up for working on the side whilst at the same time being pursued for maintenance by the Child Support Agency. I couldn't convince them, because they saw me just as an *absent father*, who was disgruntled and would say anything, and, erm, they, the Child Support Agency, although I had four step-children, dismissed [names step-children with Carolyn] and said that they, and they actually wrote to us … They said, "They do not count, you are an absent parent." It meant [current partner] was worse off and her children were worse off than before I moved in, and I thought that was intolerable.' (Victor, age 44, re-partnered father (IGE))

The effects of care responsibilities and constraint on men's well being; emotional responses

Despite wanting the best for their children and grandchildren, the balancing of care needs and responsibilities alongside additional external pressures from those that intervene in their lives can be a struggle for these men and they talk a lot about trying to control their emotions. The daily struggle of finding money to care for young children is also a problem for the younger men and affects finances when parenting. Older men are more at risk of experiencing breakdowns under the pressure of providing care at the expense of being able to work. They require support to manage the emotions that arise from difficult circumstances.

'Every day, all the time. All we ever do is struggle. But we figure a way out ... I'd like to be able to say when he asks for stuff "oh yes you can have it". But most the time I've gotta say "right, you'll have to wait until we've got enough money".' (Darren, age 21, in a relationship, receiving welfare benefits (FYF))

'I mean I'm quick tempered, don't get me wrong I'm very quick tempered because me dad were same but like, say if [granddaughter] started and all that I have to walk away. Cos I know I've told her many times I have to walk away and it's hard, it's a hard thing to do walking away, you know what I mean? A little kid's having a go at you and it's, it's hard, your own grandkid's having a go at you ... It's hard thing to walk away, it is [laughs] you know what I mean, it's, it's very hard I find it difficult you know ...

'This is the hard part I can't get, get me head round, you know what I mean. This is the worst part for me because like [third sector practitioner] said I've worked all me life and like I say I had to give a good job up financially. I couldn't take it, there were so much pressure on me.' (Geoff, age 59, kinship carer, in care as a child (IGE))

'[In maternal grandparents care] [son]'s been found to have some bruising on his leg ... it's ... we've gone to a paediatrician to see, find out if it's non-accidental or anything ... and they've ruled out that it, it's not an accident, someone's done it deliberately. But I'd rather not think like that. So, but upsetting. So he's back on the child protection plan again which, which was established yesterday. So [his mum] reported it to the social worker who then reported it to, well no I didn't get, I didn't get found out until the next day cos I'm always kept out of the loop by them ... So it's a bit, even more frustrating for me ... I've had a few times where I could have hit a wall, say.' (Adam, age 17 (FYF))

Key messages

- Men tend to be painted as dangerous or risky, yet they do play active *caregiving roles* in their families and, over time, continue to invest in caregiving.
- Care responsibilities are not limited to fathering and grandfathering. Men look out for the people in their personal networks of care and try to protect them from the trappings of their locality,
- Men do not just become 'bad dads' over time and abandon their children, as broader stereotypes such as the 'absent' and 'feckless' father would suggest. They have strong aspirations to be involved in their children's lives from a young age, and when they look back as grandfathers they relish the opportunity of a second chance to learn from their mistakes,
- Men face a number of constraints over time, however, that impact upon the extent to which they can fulfil their care responsibilities. These include:
  - negotiating sometimes difficult relationships with the mothers of their children;
  - balancing multiple responsibilities; following relationship breakdown in particular, men must make constrained choices about how they spread their resources, both financially and emotionally;
  - trying to manage the emotional consequences of negotiating care responsibilities in constrained circumstances (as separated or non-resident dads, or kinship carers);
  - lack of knowledge about rights, and dwindling financial and legal support.

New empirical project based on emerging evidence

The evidence indicates that there may be significant cumulative effects for men that influence the extent to which they can fulfil their care responsibilities. These effects may start in the men's early life and build up over the lifecourse. *We lack research on how continuing hardship and/or changing family circumstances influence the decisions men make about distributing their limited resources within their personal networks of care at different times in their lives.* This study will therefore involve looking at men's care responsibilities in low-income localities over time.

Central question of the research: How do men living on a low income define, experience and balance their care responsibilities over time?

This may break down into these areas.

1. How far do men's personal histories influence their ideas of care responsibilities and their ability to fulfil these responsibilities?
2. How far do men's personal histories shape their hopes for the future?
3. What do men think is 'good' care and what are the key barriers and constraints (perceived and actual) to them providing this care over time?
4. What do you think are the key barriers and constraints on these men?
5. How might your organisation better support men in low-income localities when they have multiple care responsibilities?

What should I add?

Whom I expect to involve in the research

- Men living in low-income localities in the north of England, who have circumstances that may be described as chaotic or 'troubled'.
- Men across all age groups with multiple care responsibilities, within and across households (fathers, grandfathers).

What should I add?

Notes

Chapter 1

[1] A delivery arm of the Department for Work and Pensions in the UK, the Child Support Agency was a child maintenance service established to implement the Child Support Act (1991). This became known as the Child Maintenance Service in 2012.

[2] The Timescapes programme of research was funded by the ESRC between 2007 and 2012 (See: https://timescapes-archive.leeds.ac.uk/timescapes/the-timescapes-initiative/). Timescapes was a large-scale, qualitative longitudinal research study carried out by a network of researchers from five universities across the UK (Leeds, London, London South Bank, The Open University and Cardiff; Holland and Edwards, 2014). The connected projects examined the dynamics of relationships, identities and family lives through the lifecourse. Through the establishment of the Timescapes Archive, concerted efforts were made to enhance the possibilities of data archiving and the reuse of qualitative longitudinal data. MPLC was one of the first funded studies to bring together and analyse data from two archived Timescapes datasets. The methods and outcomes of this work are presented in various publications (Tarrant, 2017; Hughes and Tarrant, 2019; Tarrant and Hughes, 2019).

[3] The concept of generation is contested and has several meanings (Nilsen, 2014). It is both a structural phenomenon and socially constructed. In this book it is predominantly used to refer to ties and generational identities in families.

[4] Defining the sample in terms of their differing familial identities and positions is influenced by working with the two Timescapes datasets. As analysis of the data has progressed, these categories have proved to be too deterministic to develop a fully nuanced analysis. This has resulted in a shift in analytical focus to an interpretation of the diversity of caring arrangements and family trajectories expressed across the sample.

[5] Kinship care, also known as family and friends care in the UK, is a significant feature of the placement possibilities for children who cannot live with birth parents. It is also a term used by local authorities and in official documents to define family or friends carers to children when parents can no longer provide adequate care (Grandparents Plus, 2018; Hunt, 2018).

[6] These have now been grouped together as part of the new Universal Credit system, a welfare reform intended to make the process of claiming social security more straightforward and paid monthly to reflect how people are paid in work (Millar and Bennett, 2017).

[7] https://smallprintcompany.com/

Chapter 2

[1] I explore exceptions to this later in the book, considering more recent interventions in debates about the reconciliation of work and care that consider the extent to which care might be regendered in recession and austerity contexts and open up new opportunities for men's participation in family contexts.

[2] Parenthood and family interdependencies, as key lifecourse domains, are an underexplored biographical career for those young men who become fathers at a young age.

Chapter 3

[1] These three conceptual premises are adapted from a major EU study called 'Families and Societies', funded within the EU Seventh Framework Programme (2013–2017). Its full title, 'Changing Families and Sustainable Societies: Policy Contexts and Diversity over the Life Course and Across Generations', more fully captures the broad conceptual and theoretical underpinnings that were also drivers of MPLC.

[2] In recent years these competing expectations on contemporary men have been reconceptualised in the discursive tension between 'cash and carry' (Burgess and Davies, 2017).

Chapter 4

[1] The laws around legal aid changed in 2013. For family cases it is still possible to qualify on certain grounds (for example, care cases, mediation, injunctions and child abduction, Access Law Solicitors, 2020) but it was largely believed to have been discontinued at the time.

[2] A C100 form is used to apply for a court order either to make arrangements for a child(ren) or to resolve a dispute about their upbringing.

[3] Special Guardianship Orders are a formal kinship care order that offer greater legal security and control to carers by appointing one or two people other than birth parents as 'special guardians' of a child, with day-to-day responsibility for their care.

Chapter 5

[1] The term kinship care is complex and contested. It refers to a spectrum of informal practices of caregiving across generations, as well as state-ratified and formal care arrangements that carry a certain amount of resource and state support (although this can be limited). Of the seven men interviewed as kinship carers the majority were providing kinship care informally and either had not yet acquired legal status or were in the process of securing it. This reflects the complex problem of how kinship care is constructed and defined in the UK, and that family members in low-income families are likely to engage in informal support across generations. It is usually when they need to access resources or support from the state that this becomes significant as a policy identity.

[2] While Shane is was over 25, his reflections on his circumstances are explored here for their analytic relevance. He had a partner at the time of the interview but was primarily responsible for his biological son and foster carer for his son's half- sibling.

[3] Like the participants, the children and other family members referred to in this chapter and throughout the book have been given pseudonyms to protect their identities and to enhance the readability of the narratives.

[4] These include the early death of a parent, criminal behaviour and experience of the youth offending system and mental illness.

Chapter 6

[1] The Care Act 2014 came into effect on 1 April 2015. It represents the most significant reform of care and support in over 60 years. Based on the principles and policy of personalisation, the Act is one of a suite of austerity-driven reforms that aim to address the needs of adults with care needs and of carers by giving them

greater control over their care and support. Personalisation was developed to change the nature and balance of services at a time of deepening financial challenges to public services and pressure to maintain services (ADASS, 2017).

Chapter 7

[1] References are not provided for ethical purposes, namely to protect the identity of the locality.

References

Abdill, A. (2018) *Fathering from the Margins: An Intimate Examination of Black Fatherhood.* New York: Columbia University Press.

Access Law Solicitors (2020) Breaking the myth that legal aid has been abolished, www.accesslaw.co.uk/breaking-the-myth-that-legal-aid-has-been-abolished/

Ackers, G. (2017) The impact of deindustrialisation on masculine career identity: an intergenerational study on men from naval repair families in Medway, Kent. PhD thesis: University of Huddersfield, https://researchportal.port.ac.uk/portal/files/8185798/Phd_Final.pdf

ADASS (2017) *It's Still Personal,* Directors of Adult Social Services Report, www.adass.org.uk/media/5950/its-still-personal-june-2017.pdf

Alexander, C. (1998) Re-imagining the Muslim community, *Innovation,* 11: 439–450.

Allen, K., Tyler, I. and De Benedictis, S. (2014) Thinking with 'White Dee': the gender politics of austerity porn, *Sociological Research Online,* 19 (3): 2, www.socresonline.org.uk/19/3/2.html

Allen, S. and Daly, K. (2002) *The Effects of Father Involvement: A Summary of the Research Evidence, The Father Involvement Initiative,* Volume 1, www.ecdip.org/docs/pdf/IF%20Father%20Res%20Summary%20(KD).pdf

Anderson, E. (1999) *Code of the Street: Decency, Violence, and the Moral Life of the Inner City.* New York: W.W. Norton & Company.

Anderson, E. (2009) *Inclusive Masculinity: The Changing Nature of Masculinities.* Abingdon: Routledge.

Andreasson, J. and Johansson, T. (2019) Becoming a half-time parent: Fatherhood after divorce, *Journal of Family Issues,* 25 (1): 2–17.

Arnold, J. and Brady, S. (2011) *What Is Masculinity? Historical Dynamics from Antiquity to the Contemporary World,* Basingstoke: Palgrave Macmillan.

Ashe, F. (2014) 'All about Eve': mothers, masculinities and the 2011 UK riots, *Political Studies,* 62 (3): 652–668.

Bailey, J. (2010) 'A very sensible man': imagining fatherhood in England c. 1750–1830, *History,* 95 (319): 267–292.

Baird, A. (2012) The violent gang and the construction of masculinity amongst socially excluded young men, *Safer Communities,* 11: 179–190.

Bartova, A. and Keizer, R. (2020) How well do European child-related leave policies support the caring role of fathers? In: R. Nieuwenhuis and W. Van Lancker (eds), *The Palgrave Handbook of Family Policy*. Basingstoke: Palgrave Macmillan.

Baskerville, S. (2004) Is there really a fatherhood crisis? *The Independent Review*, 8 (4): 485–508.

BBC News (2020) Knife offenders lack male role models, says senior police officer, www.bbc.co.uk/news/uk-51682870

Beck, U. and Beck-Gernsheim, E. (1995) *The Normal Chaos of Love*. Cambridge: Polity Press.

Beck, U. and Beck-Gernsheim, E. (2002) *Individualization*. London: Sage.

Bedston, S., Philip, G., Youansamouth, L., Clifton, J., Broadhurst, K., Brandon, M. and Hu, Y. (2019) Linked lives: gender, family relations and recurrent care proceedings in England, *Children and Youth Services Review*, 105: 1–13.

Beggs Weber, J. (2020) Being there (or not): teen dads, gendered age, and negotiating the absent-father discourse, *Men and Masculinities*, 23 (1): 42–64.

Ben-Galim, D. and Silim, A. (2013) *The Sandwich Generation: Older Women Balancing Work and Care*, IPPR Report, www.ippr.org/files/images/media/files/publication/2013/08/sandwich-generation-August2013_11168_11168.pdf

Bengtsson, T. and Ravn, S. (2019) *Youth, Risk, Routine: A New Perspective on Risk-Taking in Young Lives*. London: Routledge.

Bennett, F. and Daly, M. (2014) *Poverty through a Gender Lens: Evidence and Policy Review on Gender and Poverty*. York: Joseph Rowntree Foundation Report.

Bertaux, D. and Thompson, P. (1997) *Pathways to Social Class: A Qualitative Approach to Social Mobility*. Oxford: Oxford University Press.

Bjørnholt, M. (2014) Changing men, changing times – fathers and sons from an experimental gender equality study, *The Sociological Review*, 62 (2): 295–315.

Bond-Taylor, S. (2016) Domestic surveillance and the Troubled Families Programme: understanding relationality and constraint in the homes of multiply disadvantaged families, *People, Place and Policy*, 10 (3): 207–224.

Bonner-Thompson, C. and McDowell, L. (2020) Precarious lives, precarious care: young men's caring practices in three coastal towns in England, *Emotion, Space and Society*, 35: 1–7.

Boothroyd, L.G. and Perrett, D.I. (2008) Father absence, parent–daughter relationships and partner preferences, *Journal of Evolutionary Psychology*, 6 (3): 187–205.

Bottero, W. (2008) Class in the 21st century. In: Runnymede Trust (ed), *Who Cares about the White Working Class?* www.runnymedetrust.org/uploads/publications/pdfs/WhoCaresAboutTheWhiteWorkingClass-2009.pdf, 7–14.

Bowlby, S., McKie, L., Gregory, S. and MacPherson, I. (2010) *Interdependency and Care over the Life Course.* Abingdon: Routledge.

Boyer, K., Dermott, E., James, A. and MacLeavy, J. (2017) Regendering care in the aftermath of recession? *Dialogues in Human Geography*, 7 (1): 56–73.

Bradshaw, J., Stimson, C., Skinner, C. and Williams, J. (1999) *Absent Fathers?* Abingdon: Routledge.

Brah, A. and Phoenix, A. (2004) Ain't I a woman? Revisiting intersectionality, *Journal of International Women's Studies*, 5 (3): 75–86.

Brandon, M., Philip, G. and Clifton, J. (2017) 'Counting fathers in': understanding men's experiences of the child protection system, University of East Anglia Report.

Brannen, J. (2019) *Social Research Matters: A Life in Family Sociology.* Bristol: Bristol University Press.

Brannen, J. and Nilsen, A. (2006) From fatherhood to fathering: transmission and change among British fathers in four-generation families, *Sociology*, 40 (2): 335–352.

Brannen, J., Parutis, V., Mooney, A. and Wigfall, V. (2011) Fathers and intergenerational transmission in social context, *Ethics and Education*, 6 (2): 155–170.

Braun, A., Vincent, C. and Ball, S. (2011) Working-class fathers and childcare: the economic and family contexts of fathering in the UK, *Community Work and Family*, 1: 19–37.

Brooks, R. and Hodkinson, P. (2020) *Sharing Care: Equal and Primary Carer Fathers and Early Years Parenting.* Bristol: Policy Press.

Brown, L., Callahan, M., Strega, S., Walmsley, C. and Dominelli, L. (2009) Manufacturing ghost fathers: the paradox of father presence and absence in child welfare, *Child and Family Social Work*, 14 (1): 25–34.

Brown, S. (2015) Using focus groups in naturally occurring settings, *Qualitative Research Journal*, 15 (1): 86–97.

Bryson, C., Ellman, I.M., McKay, S. and Miles, J. (2015) *Child Maintenance: How Would the British Public Calculate What the State Should Require Parents to Pay?* London: Nuffield Foundation.

Buchanan, A. and Rotkirch, A. (2016) *Grandfathers: Global Perspectives.* London: Springer.

Bulman, K. and Neale, B. (2017) Developing sustained support for vulnerable young fathers: journeys with young offenders. In: A. Tarrant and B. Neale (eds) *Learning to Support Young Dads.* Responding to Young Fathers in a Different Way: Project Report.

Burgess, A. and Davies, J. (2017) *Cash or Carry? Fathers Combining Work and Care in the UK* (Full Report), Contemporary Fathers in the UK series, Marlborough: Fatherhood Institute.

Bywaters, P., Bunting, L., Davidson, G., Hanratty, J., Mason, W., McCartan, S. and Steils, N. (2016) *The Relationship Between Poverty, Child Abuse and Neglect: A Rapid Evidence Review.* London: Joseph Rowntree Foundation.

Cabrera, N., Fitzgerald, H., Bradley, R. and Roggman, L. (2014) The ecology of father–child relationships: an expanded model, *Journal of Family Theory and Review*, 6 (4): 336–354.

Calasanti, T. (2004) Feminist gerontology and old men, *Gerontology Series B*, 59 (6): 305–314.

Campbell, B. (1993) *Goliath: Britain's Dangerous Places*, London: Methuen.

Canton, J. (2018) Coping with hard times: the role that support networks play for lone mother families in times of economic crisis and government austerity, *Families, Relationships and Societies*, 7 (1): 23–38.

Carlson, M.J. and Magnuson, K.A. (2011) Low-income fathers' influence on children, *The Annals of the American Academic of Political and Social Science*, 635 (1): 95–116.

Centre for Social Justice (2013) *Fractured Families: Why Stability Matters*, www.centreforsocialjustice.org.uk/core/wp-content/uploads/2016/08/CSJ_Fractured_Families_Report_WEB_13.06.13-1.pdf

Centre for Social Justice (2016) *The Five Pathways to Poverty*, www.centreforsocialjustice.org.uk/policy/breakthrough-britain#:~:text=The%20CSJ%20is%20best%20known,as%20pathways%20to%20entrenched%20poverty

Centre for Social Justice (2017) Annual Report 2017/18, www.centreforsocialjustice.org.uk/core/wp-content/uploads/2018/10/CSJ-Annual-Report.pdf

Chambers, D. (2012) *A Sociology of Family Life.* Cambridge: Polity Press.

Charles, N. and Crow, G. (2012) Community re-studies and social change, *The Sociological Review*, 60 (3): 399–404.

Chesley, N. (2011) Stay-at-home fathers and breadwinning mothers: gender, couple dynamics, and social change, *Gender and Society*, 25 (5): 642–664.

Chung, H. and van de Lippe, T. (2021) Flexible working, work–life balance, and gender equality: introduction, *Social Indicators Research*, 151: 365-381.

Churchill, H. (2020) Children and families. In: H. Bochel and G. Daly (eds) *Social Policy* (4th edn). London: Routledge.

Coffield, F., Robinson, P. and Sarsby, J. (1980) *A Cycle of Deprivation? A Case of Four Families*, Portsmouth: Heineman Educational.

Cohen, S. (2002) *Folk Devils and Moral Panics: The Creation of the Mods and Rockers*. London: Routledge.

Collier, R. (1998) *Masculinities, Crime and Criminology: Men, Heterosexuality and the Criminal(ised) Other*. London: Sage.

Collier, R. and Sheldon, S. (2008) *Fragmenting Fatherhood: A Socio-Legal Study*. Oxford: Hart Publishing.

Comas-d'Argemir, D. and Soronellas, M. (2019) Men as carers in long-term caring: doing gender and doing kinship, *Journal of Family Issues*, 40 (3): 315–339.

Conlon, C., Timonen, V., Carney, G. and Scharf, T. (2014) Women (re)negotiating care across family generations: intersections of gender and socioeconomic status, *Gender and Society*, 28 (5): 729–751.

Connell, R.W. (1995) *Masculinities*. Cambridge, MA: California University Press.

Connell, R.W. (2001) Introduction and overview. Special issue on men and masculinities: discursive approaches, *Feminism and Psychology*, 11: 5–9.

Connell, R.W. (2010) Lives of the businessmen: reflections on life-history method and contemporary hegemonic masculinity, *Österreichische Zeitschrift für Soziologie*, 35 (2): 54–71.

Connell, R.W. and Messerschmidt, J. (2005) Hegemonic masculinity: rethinking the concept, *Gender and Society*, 19 (6): 829–859.

Cooper, K. (2013) Revealing the lived reality of kinship care through children and young people's narratives: 'It's not all nice, it's not all easy-going, it's a difficult journey to go on'. In: J. Ribbens McCarthy, V. Gillies and C.-A. Hooper (eds). *Family Troubles? Exploring Changes and Challenges in the Family Lives of Children and Young People*. Bristol: Policy Press.

Crenshaw, K. (1989) Demarginalizing the intersection of race and sex: a black feminist critique of antidiscrimination doctrine, feminist theory and antiracist politics, *University of Chicago Legal Forum*, 140: 139–167.

Crossley, S. (2017) *In Their Place: The Imagined Geographies of Poverty*. London: Pluto Press.

Crow, G. (2002) *Social Solidarities: Theories, Identities and Social Change.* Buckingham: Open University Press.

Cunningham-Burley, S. (1984) 'We don't talk about it …': issues of gender and method in the portrayal of grandfatherhood, *Sociology*, 18 (3): 325–338.

Daly, K.J. (1996) Spending time with the kids: meanings of family time for fathers, *Family Relations*, 45 (4): 466–476.

Daly, M. (2018) Towards a theorization of the relationship between poverty and family, *Social Policy and Administration*, 52 (3): 565–577.

Daly, M. and Kelly, G. (2015) *Families and Poverty: Everyday Life on a Low Income.* Bristol: Policy Press.

Daly, M. and Lewis, J. (2000) The concept of social care and the analysis of contemporary welfare states, *British Journal of Sociology*, 51: 281–298.

Daly, M. and Rake, K. (2003) *Gender and the Welfare State.* Oxford: Polity Marketing.

Daniels, C.R. (1998) *Lost Fathers: The Politics of Fatherlessness in America.* New York: St Martin's Griffin.

Davis, A. and King, L. (2018) Gendered perspectives on men's changing familial roles in postwar England, c. 1950–1990, *Gender and History*, 30 (1): 70–92.

De Benedictis, S. (2012) Feral parents: austerity parenting under neoliberalism, *Studies in the Maternal*, 4 (2): 1–21.

Delgado, M. (2015) *Urban Youth and Photovoice: Visual Ethnography in Action.* Oxford: Oxford University Press.

Demey, D., Berrington, A., Evandrou, M. and Falkingham, J. (2013) Pathways into living alone in mid-life: diversity and policy implications, *Advances in Life Course Research*, 18 (3): 161–174.

Dennis, N. and Erdos, G. (1992) *Families without Fatherhood.* Wiltshire: The Cromwell Press.

Department for Work and Pensions (2018) *Economic Labour Market Status of Individuals Aged 50 and over, Trends over Time: September 2019*, https://assets.publishing.service.gov.uk/government/uploads/system/uploads/attachment_data/file/830825/economic-labour-market-status-of-individuals-aged-50-and-over-sept-2019.pdf

Dermott, E. (2003) The 'intimate father': defining paternal involvement, *Sociological Research Online*, 8 (4), www.socresonline.org.uk/8/4/dermott.html

Dermott, E. (2008) *Intimate Fatherhood: A Sociological Analysis* (2nd edn). Abingdon: Routledge.

Dermott, E. (2016) Non-resident fathers in the UK: living standards and social support, *Journal of Poverty and Social Justice*, 24 (2): 113–125.

Dermott, E. and Gatrell, C. (2018) *Fathers, Families and Relationships: Researching Everyday* Lives. Bristol: Bristol University Press.

Dermott, E. and Miller, T. (2015) More than the sum of its parts? Contemporary fatherhood policy, practice and discourse, *Families, Relationships and Societies*, 4 (2): 183–195.

Dermott, E. and Pantazis, C. (2014) Gender and poverty in Britain: changes and continuities between 1999 and 2012, *Journal of Poverty and Social Justice*, 22 (3): 253–269.

Dermott, E. and Pomati, M. (2016) 'Good' parenting practices: how important are poverty, education and time pressure? *Sociology*, 50 (1): 125–142.

Desmond, M. (2012) Disposable ties and the urban poor, *American Journal of Sociology*, 117 (5): 1295–1335.

Deuchar, R. (2009) *Gangs, Marginalised Youth and Social Capital*. Stoke-on-Trent: Trentham Books.

Deutsch, F.M. and Gaunt, R.A. (2020) *Creating Equality at Home: How 25 Couples around the World Share Housework and Childcare*. Cambridge: Cambridge University Press.

Dicks, B., Waddington, D. and Critcher, C. (1998) Redundant men and overburdened women: local service providers and the construction of gender in ex-mining communities. In: J. Popay, J. Hearn and J. Edwards (eds), *Men, Gender Divisions and Welfare*. Abingdon: Routledge. 287–311.

Dolan, A. (2014) 'I've learnt what a dad should do': the interaction of masculine and fathering identities among men who attended a 'dads only' parenting programme, *Sociology*, 48 (4): 812–828.

Doucet, A. (2011) 'It's just not good for a man to be interested in other people's children': fathers, public displays of care and 'relevant others'. In: E. Dermott and J. Seymour (eds), *Displaying Families*. Basingstoke: Palgrave Macmillan, 81–110.

Doucet, A. (2017) The ethics of care and the radical potential of fathers 'home alone on leave': care as practice, relational ontology, and social justice. In: M. O'Brien and K. Wall (eds), *Comparative Perspectives on Work-Life Balance and Gender Equality*. London: Springer International Publishing.

Doucet, A. (2018) *Do Men Mother? Fathering, Care and Paternal Responsibilities* (2nd edn). Toronto: University of Toronto Press.

Doucet, A. (2020) Father involvement, care, and breadwinning: genealogies of concepts and revisioned conceptual narratives, *Genealogy*, 4 (1): 14.

Du Bois, W.E.B. (1996 [1899]) *The Philadelphia Negro: A Social Study*, Philadelphia: University of Pennsylvania Press.

Duncan, S. (2010) What's the problem with teenage parents? And what's the problem with policy? *Critical Social Policy*, 27 (3): 307–334.

Duncan, S. and Phillips, M. (2010) People who live apart together (LATs) – how different are they? *The Sociological Review*, 58 (1): 112–134.

Dykstra, P. and Hagestad, G.O. (2007) Childlessness and parenthood in two centuries: different roads – different maps? *Journal of Family Issues*, 28 (11): 1518–1532.

Earley, V.S. (2017) Fathers in Everyday Family Life: Qualitative Case Studies of Ten Families. PhD thesis, University of Sheffield.

Edin, K. and Kissane, R.J. (2010) Poverty and the American family: a decade in review, *Journal of Marriage and Family*, 72(3), 460–479.

Edin, K. and Nelson, T.J. (2013) *Doing the Best I Can: Fatherhood in the Inner City*. Berkeley: University of California Press.

Edwards, R. and Gillies, V. (2012) Farewell to family? Notes on an argument for retaining the concept, *Families, Relationships and Societies*, 1 (1): 63–69.

Edwards, R. and Irwin, S. (2010) Lived experience through economic downturn in Britain – perspectives across time and across the lifecourse, *Twenty-first Century Society*, 5 (2): 119–124.

Edwards, R., Gillies, V. and Horsley, N. (2015) Brain science and early years policy: hopeful ethos or 'cruel optimism'? *Critical Social Policy*, 35 (2): 167–187.

Eisenstadt, N. and Oppenheim, C. (2019) *Parents, Poverty and the State: 20 Years of Evolving Family Policy*. Bristol: Policy Press.

Elder, Jr., G.H. (1994) Time, human agency, and social change: perspectives on the life course, *Social Psychology Quarterly*, 57 (1): 4–15.

Elder, Jr., G.H. and Giele, J.Z. (2009) Life course studies: an evolving field. In: G.H. Elder, Jr and J.Z. Giele (eds), *The Craft of Life Course Research*. New York: The Guilford Press, 1–24.

Elliott, K. (2016) Caring masculinities: theorizing an emerging concept, *Men and Masculinities*, 19 (3): 240–259.

Elliott, K. (2020) Bringing in margin and centre: 'open' and 'closed' as concepts for considering men and masculinities, *Gender, Place and Culture*, 27 (12): 1723–1744.

Emmel, N. (2017) Empowerment in the relational longitudinal space of vulnerability, *Social Policy and Society*, 16 (3): 457–467.

Emmel, N. and Hughes, K. (2010) 'Recession, it's all the same to us son': the longitudinal experience (1999–2010) of deprivation, *Twenty-First Century Society*, 5(2): 171–181.

Emmel, N. and Hughes, K. (2014) Vulnerability, intergenerational exchange and the conscience of generations. In: R. Edwards and J. Holland (eds), *Understanding Families over Time: Research and Policy*. Basingstoke: Palgrave Macmillan.

Emmel, N., Hughes, K., Greenhalgh, J. and Sales, A. (2007) Accessing socially excluded people – trust and the gatekeeper in the researcher–participant relationship, *Sociological Research Online*, 12 (2): 43–55.

Enderstein, A.M. and Boonzaier, F. (2015) Narratives of young South African fathers: redefining masculinity through fatherhood, *Journal of Gender Studies*, 24 (5): 512–527.

Fatherhood Institute (2010) *Fatherhood Institute Research Summary: African Caribbean Fathers*, www.fatherhoodinstitute.org/2010/fatherhood-institute-research-summary-african-caribbean-fathers/

Fatherhood Institute (2013) *Fatherhood Institute Research Summary: Young Fathers*, www.fatherhoodinstitute.org/2013/fatherhood-institute-research-summary-young-fathers/

Featherstone, B. (2003) Taking fathers seriously, *The British Journal of Social Work*, 33 (1): 239–254.

Featherstone, B. (2009) *Contemporary Fathering: Theory, Policy and Practice*. Bristol: Policy Press.

Featherstone, B. (2013) Working with fathers: risk or resource. In: J. Ribbens McCarthy, V. Gillies and C.-A. Hooper (eds), *Family Troubles? Exploring Changes and Challenges in the Family Lives of Children and Young People*. Bristol: Policy Press.

Featherstone, B., Robb, M., Ruxton, S. and Ward, M.R. (2017) 'They are just good people … generally good people': perspectives of young men on relationships with social care workers in the UK, *Children and Society*, 31 (5): 331–341.

Finch, J. (2007) Displaying families, *Sociology*, 41 (1): 65–81.

Finch, J. and Groves, D. (1983) *A Labour of Love: Women, Work and Caring*. London: Routledge.

Finch, J. and Mason, J. (1993) *Negotiating Family Responsibilities*. London: Routledge.

Fink, J. and Lomax, H. (2014) Challenging images? Dominant, residual and emergent meanings in on-line media representations of child poverty, *Journal for the Study of British Cultures*, 21 (1): 79–95.

Fluri, J.L. and Piedalue, A. (2017) Embodying violence: critical geographies of gender, race, and culture, *Gender, Place and Culture*, 24 (4): 534–544.

Fodor, E. (2006) A different type of gender gap: how women and men experience poverty, *East European Politics and Societies*, 20 (1): 14–39.

Fox, B. (2009) *When Couples Become Parents: The Creation of Gender in the Transition to Parenthood.* Toronto: University of Toronto Press.

Fox Harding, L. (1991) *Perspectives in Child Care Policy.* London: Routledge.

Fraser, A. (2015) *Urban Legends.* Oxford: Oxford University Press.

Freeman, T. (2003) Loving fathers or deadbeat dads: the crisis of fatherhood in popular culture. In: S. Earle (eds) *Gender, Identity and Reproduction.* Basingstoke: Palgrave Macmillan, 33–49.

Furstenberg, F.F., Jr (1998) Social capital and the role of fathers in the family. In: A. Booth and A.C. Crouter (eds) *Men in Families: When Do They Get Involved? What Difference Does It Make?* Marwah, NJ: Lawrence Erlbaum Associates Publishers, 295–301.

Gatrell, C.J., Burnett, S.B., Cooper, C.L. and Sparrow, P. (2015) The price of love: the prioritisation of childcare and income earning among UK fathers, *Families, Relationships and Societies,* 4 (2): 225–238.

Genest Dufault, S. and Castelain Meunier, C. (2017) Masculinities and families in transformation, *Enfances, Familles, Generations,* 26.

Ghate, D. and Hazel, N. (2002) *Parenting in Poor Environments: Stress, Support and Coping.* New York: Jessica Kingsley Publishers.

Giddens, A. (1991) *Modernity and Self-Identity: Self and Society in the Late Modern Age.* Cambridge: Polity Press.

Gillies, V. (2003) *Family and Intimate Relationships: A Review of the Sociological Research,* Families and Social Capital ESRC Research Group Working Paper No 2.

Gillies, V. (2007) *Marginalised Mothers: Exploring Working Class Experiences of Parenting.* Abingdon: Routledge.

Gillies, V. (2009) Understandings and experiences of involved fathering in the United Kingdom: exploring classed dimensions, *Annals of the American Academy of Political and Social Science,* 624 (1): 49–60.

Gillies, V. and Edwards, R. (2005) Secondary analysis in exploring family and social change: addressing the issue of context, *FORUM: Qualitative Social Research,* 6 (1): Art 44.

Gilligan, C. (1982) *In a Different Voice.* Cambridge, MA: Harvard University Press.

Glenn, E.N. (2010) *Forced to Care: Coercion and Caregiving.* Cambridge, MA: Harvard University Press.

Goldman, R. and Burgess, A. (2017) *Where's the Daddy? Fathers and Father Figures in UK Datasets,* Contemporary Fathers in the UK series. Marlborough: Fatherhood Institute.

Goode, J. (2010) The role of gender dynamics in decisions on credit and debt in low income families, *Critical Social Policy,* 30 (1): 99–119.

Goode, J. (2012) Brothers are doing it for themselves? Men's experiences of getting into and getting out of debt, *The Journal of Socio-Economics*, 41 (3): 327–335.

Goode, J. and Waring, A. (2011) *Seeking Direction: Men, Money Advice and the Road to Financial Health*. London: Money Advice Trust.

Grandparents Plus (2018) What is Kinship Care? https://kinship.org.uk/for-kinship-carers/what-is-kinship-care/

Gray, J., Geraghty, R. and Ralph, D. (2016) *Family Rhythms: The Changing Textures of Family Life in Ireland*. Manchester: Manchester University Press.

Greer Murphy, A. (2019) Mothers in austerity. In: C. Bambra (ed), *Health in Hard Times: Austerity and Health Inequalities*. Bristol: Policy Press.

Gunter, A. (2010) *Growing Up Bad: Black Youth, Road Culture and Badness in an East London Neighbourhood*. London: Tufnell Press.

Gunter, A. and Watt, P. (2009) Grafting, going to college and working on road: youth transitions and cultures in an East London neighbourhood, *Journal of Youth Studies*, 12 (5): 515–529.

Hadley, R.A. and Hanley, T.S. (2011) Involuntary childless men and the desire for fatherhood, *Journal of Reproductive and Infant Psychology*, 29 (1): 56–68.

Hakovirta, M. (2011) Child maintenance and child poverty: a comparative analysis, *Journal of Poverty and Social Justice*, 19 (3): 249–262.

Hall, S.M. (2016a) Everyday family experiences of the financial crisis: getting by in the recent economic recession, *Journal of Economic Geography*, 16 (2): 305–330.

Hall, S.M. (2016b) Families, intergenerationality, and peer group relations. In: S. Punch and R. Vanderbeck (eds), *Geographies of Children and Young People*. London: Springer Nature.

Hall, S.M. (2019) *Everyday Life in Austerity: Family, Friends and Intimate Relations*. Basingstoke: Palgrave Macmillan.

Hall, S.M. and Hiteva, R. (2020) Introduction. In: S.M. Hall and R. Hiteva (eds), *Engaging with Policy, Practice and Publics: Intersectionality and Impact*. Bristol: Policy Press.

Hall, S.M., Leary, K. and Greevy, H. (2014) *Public Attitudes to Poverty*. York: Joseph Rowntree Foundation.

Hanlon, N. (2012) *Masculinities, Care and Equality: Identity and Nurture in Men's Lives*. Basingstoke: Palgrave Macmillan.

Hanna, E. (2018) *Supporting Young Men as Fathers: Gendered Understandings of Group-based Community Provisions*. Basingstoke: Palgrave Macmillan.

Harker, C. and Martin, L. (2012) Familial relations: spaces, subjects, and politics, *Environment and Planning A: Economy and Space*, 44 (4): 768–775.

Haywood, C. and Johansson, T. (2017) *Marginalized Masculinities: Contexts, Continuities and Change.* London: Routledge.

Hearn, J. (1998) Troubled masculinities in social policy discourses: young men. In: J. Popay, J. Hearn and J. Edwards (eds), *Men, Gender Divisions and Welfare.* London: Routledge.

Hebdige, D. (1988) *Hiding in the Light.* London: Comedia.

Hemmerman, L. (2010) *Researching the Hard to Reach and the Hard to Keep: Notes from the Field on Longitudinal Sample Maintenance,* Timescapes Working Paper Series No 2, www.timescapes.leeds. ac.uk/assets/files/WP2-final-Jan-2010.pdf

Henwood, K. and Procter, J. (2003) The 'good father': reading men's accounts of paternal involvement during the transition to first-time fatherhood, *British Journal of Psychology,* 42 (3): 337–355.

Henwood, K., Shirani, F. and Coltart, C. (2010) Fathers and financial risk-taking during the economic downturn: insights from a QLL study of men's identities-in-the-making, *Twenty-First Century Society,* 5 (2): 137–147.

Herlofson, K. and Hagestad, G.O. (2012) Transformation in the role of grandparents across welfare states. In: S. Arber and V. Timonen (eds), *Contemporary Grandparenting: Changing Family Relationships in Global Contexts.* Bristol: Policy Press.

Heward, C. (1996) Masculinities and families. In: M. Mac an Ghaill and C. Haywood (eds), *Understanding Masculinities: Social Relations and Cultural Arenas.* Buckingham: Open University Press, 35–49.

Hochschild, A. (1989) *Second Shift: Working Families and the Revolution at Home.* New York: Viking.

Hockey, J. and James, A. (2003) *Social Identities across the Lifecourse.* London: Springer.

Hogarth, T., Owen, D., Gambin, L., Hasluck, C., Lyonette, C. and Casey, B. (2009) *The Equality Impacts of the Current Recession,* Equality and Human Rights Commission Research Report Series.

Holland, J. and Edwards, R. (2014) *Introduction to Timescapes: Changing Relationships and Identities over Time.* Basingstoke: Palgrave Macmillan.

Hollway, W. (2006) *The Capacity to Care: Gender and Ethical Subjectivities.* London: Routledge.

Holmes, M. (2006) Love lives at a distance: distance relationships over the lifecourse, *Sociological Research Online,* 11 (3): 70–80.

hooks, b. (2004) *The Will to Change: Men, Masculinity, and Love.* New York: Beyond Words/Atria Books.

Hopkins, P. (2006) Youthful Muslim masculinities: gender and generational relations, *Transactions of the Institute of British Geographers,* 31 (3): 337–352.

Hopkins, P. (2019) Social geography I: intersectionality, *Progress in Human Geography*, 43 (5): 937–947.

Hopkins, P. and Noble, G. (2009) Masculinities in place: situated identities, relations and intersectionality, *Social and Cultural Geography*, 10: 811–819.

Hopkins, P. and Pain, R. (2007) Geographies of age: thinking relationally, *Area*, 39 (3): 287–294.

Horsley, N., Gillies, V. and Edwards, R. (2020) 'We've got a file on you': problematising families in poverty in four periods of austerity, *Journal of Poverty and Social Justice*, 28 (2): 227–244.

Hrženjak, M. (2017) A qualitative study of labour market precarisation and involved fatherhood in Slovenia, *Revija za Sociologiju*, 47 (2): 207–232.

Hughes, K. and Emmel, N. (2011) Intergenerational exchange: grandparents, their grandchildren, and the texture of poverty. Timescapes Policy Briefing Paper Series, University of Leeds, www.timescapes.leeds.ac.uk/assets/files/Policy-Conference-2011/paper-6.pdf

Hughes, K. and Tarrant, A. (2019) *Qualitative Secondary Analysis*. London: Sage.

Hunt, J. (2018) Grandparents as substitute parents in the UK, *Contemporary Social Science*, 13 (2): 175–186.

Hunt, J. and Waterhouse, S. (2012) *Understanding Family and Friends Care: The Relationship between Need, Support and Legal Status. Carer's Experiences*. London: Family Rights Group.

Hutchison, E. (2019) An update on the relevance of the life course perspective for social work, *Families in Society: The Journal of Contemporary Social Services*, 100 (4): 351–366.

Jamieson, L. (1998) *Intimacy: Personal Relationships in Modern Societies*. Cambridge: Polity Press.

Jensen, T. (2018) *Parenting the Crisis: The Cultural Politics of Parent-Blame*. Bristol: Policy Press.

Jensen, T. and Tyler, I. (2012) Austerity parenting: new economies of parent-citizenship, *Studies in the Maternal*, 4 (2): 1.

Jensen, T. and Tyler, I. (2015) 'Benefits broods': the cultural and political crafting of anti-welfare commonsense, *Critical Social Policy*, 35 (4): 470–491.

Johansson, T. and Andreasson, J. (2018) *Fatherhood in Transition: Masculinity, Identity and Everyday Life*. Basingstoke: Palgrave MacMillan.

Jordan, A. (2020a) *The New Politics of Fatherhood: Men's Movements and Masculinities*. Basingstoke: Palgrave Macmillan.

Jordan, A. (2020b) Masculinizing care? Gender, ethics of care, and fathers' rights groups, *Men and Masculinities*, 23 (1): 20–41.

Jordan, A. and Chandler, A. (2019) Crisis, what crisis? A feminist analysis of discourse on masculinities and suicide, *Journal of Gender Studies*, 28 (4): 462–474.

Jupp, E. (2017) Families, policy and place in times of austerity, *Area*, 49 (3): 266–272.

Katz, I., Corylon, J., La Placa, V. and Hunter, S. (2007) *The Relationship between Parenting and Poverty*. York: Joseph Rowntree Foundation.

Keating, N., Eales, J., Funk, L., Fast, J. and Min, J. (2019) Life course trajectories of family care, *International Journal of Care and Caring*, 3 (2): 147–163.

Kemp, P.A., Bradshaw, J., Dornan, P., Finch, N. and Mayhew, E. (2004) *Routes out of Poverty: A Research Review*. York: Joseph Rowntree Foundation.

Kilkey, M. and Clarke, H. (2010) Disabled men and fathering: opportunities and constraints, *Community, Work and Family*, 13 (2): 127–146.

King, L. (2013) 'Now you see a great many men pushing their pram proudly': family-orientated masculinity represented and experienced in mid-twentieth-century Britain, *Cultural and Social History*, 10 (4): 599–617.

King, L. (2015) *Family Men: Fatherhood and Masculinity in Britain, c. 1914–1960*. Oxford: Oxford University Press.

King, N. and Calasanti, T. (2013) Men's aging amidst intersecting relations of inequality, *Sociology Compass*, 7 (9): 699–710.

Kitchen, M., Martin, R. and Tyler, P. (2011) The geographies of austerity, *Cambridge Journal of Regions, Economy and Society*, 4: 289–302.

Klett-Davies, M. (2007) *Going It Alone? Lone Motherhood in Later Modernity*. Aldershot: Ashgate.

Klett-Davies, M. (2010) *Is Parenting a Class Issue?* London: Family and Parenting Institute.

Kröger, T. and Sipilä, J. (2005). *Overstretched: European Families up against the Demands of Work and Care*. Oxford: Blackwell.

Ladlow, L. and Neale, B. (2016) Rick, resource, redemption? The parenting and custodial experiences of young offender fathers, *Social Policy and Society*, 15 (1): 113–127.

Lamb, M.E. (2000) The history of research on father involvement: an overview, *Marriage and Family Review*, 29 (2/3): 23–42.

Lamb, M.E. (2010) How do fathers influence children's development? Let me count the ways. In: M.E. Lamb (ed), *The Role of the Father in Child Development*, Hoboken, NJ: Wiley.

Lambert, M. and Crossley, S. (2018) 'Getting with the (troubled families) programme': a review, *Social Policy and Society*, 16 (1): 87–97.

Lammy, D. (2011) *Out of the Ashes: Britain after the Riots*. London: Guardian Books.

Laqueur, T.W. (1990) The facts of fatherhood. In: E. Fox-Keller and M. Hirsch (eds) *Debates in Feminism*, New York: Routledge, 155–175.

LaRossa, R. (2012) The historical study of fatherhood: theoretical and methodological considerations. In: M. Oechsle, U. Muller and S. Hess (eds), *Fatherhood in Late Modernity: Cultural Images, Social Practices, Structural Frames*. Leverkusen: Barbara Budrich Publishers, 37–58.

Lee, K. (2008) Fragmenting Fatherhoods? Fathers, Fathering and Family Diversity. Unpublished doctoral thesis, City University London.

Levtov, R., van der Gaag, N., Greene, M., Kaufman, M. and Barker, G. (2015) *State of the World's Fathers*, www.savethechildren.net/sites/default/files/libraries/state-of-the-worlds-fathers_12-june-2015.pdf

Lister, R. (1996) In search of the underclass. In: *Charles Murray and the Underclass: The Developing Debate*, IEA Health and Welfare Unit, No 33, www.civitas.org.uk/pdf/cw33.pdf

MacDonald, R. (1997) *Youth, the 'Underclass' and Social Exclusion*. London: Routledge.

MacDonald, R. (2016) Voodoo sociology, unemployment and 'the low-pay, no-pay' cycle, *The SARF blog*, www.the-sarf.org.uk/voodoo-sociology/?LMCL=RynI3A

MacDonald, R. and Marsh, J. (2002) Crossing the Rubicon: youth transitions, poverty, drugs and social exclusion, *International Journal of Drug Policy*, 13 (1): 27–38.

MacDonald, R. and Shildrick, T. (2007) Biographies of exclusion: poor work and poor transitions, *International Journal of Lifelong Education*, 26 (5): 589–604.

MacDonald, R. and Shildrick, T. (2018) Biography, history and place: understanding youth transitions in Teesside. In: S. Irwin and A. Nilsen (eds), *Transitions to Adulthood Through Recession: Youth and Inequality in a European Comparative Perspective*. Abingdon: Routledge.

MacDonald, R., Shildrick, T., Webster, C. and Simpson, D. (2005) Growing up in poor neighbourhoods: significance of class and place in the extended transitions of 'socially excluded' young adults, *Sociology*, 39 (5): 873–891.

MacDonald, R., Shildrick, T. and Furlong, A. (2014) In search of intergenerational cultures of worklessness: hunting the Yeti and shooting zombies, *Critical Social Policy*, 34 (2): 199–220.

MacDonald, R., Shildrick, T. and Furlong, A. (2020) 'Cycles of disadvantage' revisited: young people, families and poverty across generations, *Journal of Youth Studies*, 23 (1): 12–27.

MacLeavy, J. (2011) A 'new politics' of austerity, workfare and gender? The UK coalition government's welfare reform proposals, *Cambridge Journal of Regions, Economy and Society*, 4 (3): 335–367.

Macnicol, J. (1987) In pursuit of the underclass, *Journal of Social Policy*, 16 (3): 293–318.

Madhavan, S., Townsend, N. and Garey, A. (2010) 'Absent-breadwinners': father–child connections and paternal support in Rural South Africa, *Journal of South African Studies*, 34 (3): 647–663.

Maguire, D. (2020) *Male, Failed, Jailed: Masculinities and 'Revolving-Door' Imprisonment in the UK*, Basingstoke: Palgrave Macmillan.

Mahadevan, J. (2011) Riots blamed on absent fathers and poor school discipline, *Children and Young People Now*, www.cypnow.co.uk/cyp/news/1049472/riots-blamed-absent-fathers-poor-school-discipline

Majors, R. (1998) Cool pose: Black masculinity and sports. In: G. Sailes (ed), *African Americans in Sport*. London: Routledge, 15–22.

Mann, K. and Roseneil, S. (1994) 'Some mothers do 'ave 'em': backlash and the gender politics of the underclass debate, *Gender and Society*, 3 (3): 317–331.

Mann, R., Tarrant, A. and Leeson, G. (2016) Grandfatherhood: shifting masculinities in later life, *Sociology*, 50 (3): 594–610.

Marriage Foundation (2018) Government under pressure to back marriage as cost of family breakdown hits £51 billion, https://marriagefoundation.org.uk/government-pressure-back-marriage-cost-family-breakdown-hits-51-billion/

Mason, J., May, V. and Clarke, L. (2007) Ambivalence and the paradoxes of grandparenting, *The Sociological Review*, 55 (4): 687–706.

Mavungu Eddy, M., Thomson-de Boor, H. and Mphaka, K. (2013) *'So we are ATM fathers': A Study of Absent Fathers in Johannesburg, South Africa*, Centre for Social Development in South Africa, www.uj.ac.za/faculties/humanities/csda/Documents/Absent-fathers-full-report%202013.pdf

Maxwell, K.J. (2018) Fatherhood in the Context of Social Disadvantage: Constructions of Fatherhood and Attitudes Towards Parenting Interventions of Disadvantaged Men in Scotland. PhD thesis, University of Glasgow.

Maxwell, N., Scourfield, J., Featherstone, B., Holland, S. and Tolman, R. (2012) Engaging fathers in child welfare services: a narrative review of recent research evidence, *Child and Family Social Work*, 17 (2): 160–169.

McCulloch, D. (2018) *Understanding Poverty Using Visual Participatory Methods: Can It Work?* ESRC National Centre for Research Methods.

McDowell, L. (2000) The trouble with men? Young people, gender transformations and the crisis of masculinity, *International Journal of Urban and Regional Research*, 4 (1): 201–209.

McDowell, L. (2002) Masculine discourses and dissonances: strutting 'lads', protest masculinity, and domestic respectability, *Environment and Planning D: Society and Space*, 20 (1): 97–119.

McDowell, L. (2003) Masculine identities and low paid work: young men in urban labour markets, *International Journal of Urban and Regional Research*, 27 (4): 828–848.

McDowell, L. (2004) Work, workfare, work/life balance and an ethic of care, *Progress in Human Geography*, 28 (2): 145–163.

McDowell, L. (2012) Post-crisis, post-Ford and post-gender? Youth identities in an era of austerity, *Journal of Youth Studies*, 15: 573–590.

McDowell, L. (2014) The sexual contract, youth, masculinity and the uncertain promise of waged work in austerity Britain, *Australian Feminist Studies*, 29 (79): 31–49.

McDowell, L. (2017) Youth, children and families in austere times: change, politics and a new gender contract, *Area*, 49 (3): 311–316.

McDowell, L., Rootham, E. and Hardgrove, A. (2014) Precarious work, protest masculinity and communal regulation: South Asian young men in Luton, UK, *Work Employment and Society*, 28 (6): 847–864.

McHardy, F. (2016) *Bairns Come First, Fairness for Their Future: A Study of Child Maintenance in Fife*, The Poverty Alliance Report.

McKay, A., Campbell, J., Thomson, E. and Ross, S. (2013) Economic recession and recovery in the UK: what's gender got to do with it? *Feminist Economics*, 19 (3): 108–123.

McKendrick, J.H., Cunningham-Burley, S. and Backett-Milburn, K. (2003) *Life in Low Income Families in Scotland: A Review of the Literature*. Edinburgh: Scottish Executive.

McKenzie, L. (2010) *Getting By: Estates, Class and Culture in Austerity Britain*. Bristol: Policy Press.

McLanahan, S., Tach, L. and Schneider, D. (2013) The causal effects of father absence, *Annual Reviews*, 39: 399–427.

Meah, A. and Jackson, P. (2016) The complex landscape of contemporary fathering in the UK, *Social and Cultural Geography*, 17 (4): 491–510.

Millar, J. and Bennett, F. (2017) Universal Credit: assumptions, contradictions and virtual reality, *Social Policy and Society*, 16 (2): 169–182.

Millar, J. and Ridge, T. (2009) Relationships of care: working lone mothers, their children and employment sustainability, *Journal of Social Policy*, 38 (1): 103–121.

Miller, T. (2010a) *Making Sense of Fatherhood: Gender, Caring and Work.* Cambridge: Cambridge University Press.

Miller, T. (2010b) Falling back into gender? Men's narratives and practices around first time fatherhood, *Sociology*, 45: 1094–1109.

Miller, T. (2018a) Paternal and maternal gatekeeping? Choreographing care, *Sociologica, International Journal for Sociological Debate*, 12 (3): 25–35.

Miller, T. (2018b) Qualitative longitudinal research: researching fatherhood and fathers' experiences. In: E. Dermott and C. Gatrell (eds), *Fathers, Families and Relationships: Researching Everyday Lives.* Bristol: Bristol University Press, pp 31–46.

Milligan, C. and Morbey, H. (2016) Care, coping and identity: older men's experiences of spousal care-giving, *Journal of Aging Studies*, 38: 105–114.

Mills, C-W. (1959) *The Sociological Imagination*, Oxford: Oxford University Press.

Mincy, R.B., Jethwani, M. and Klempin, S. (2015) *Failing Our Fathers: Confronting the Crisis of Economically Vulnerable Fathers.* Oxford: Oxford University Press.

Mitchell, W. (2007) Research review: the role of grandparents in intergenerational support for families with disable children: a review of the literature, *Child and Family Social Work*, 12: 94–101.

Morgan, D. (1996) *Family Connections: An Introduction to Family Studies.* Cambridge: Polity.

Morgan, D. (2003) The crisis of masculinity. In: K. Davis, M. Evans and J. Lorber (eds), *Handbook of Gender and Women's Studies.* London: Sage: 109–124.

Morgan, D. (2011) Locating family practices, *Sociological Research Online*, 16 (4): 14.

Morrell, R. (2016) Fathers, fatherhood and masculinity in South Africa. In: L. Richter and R. Morrell (eds), *BABA: Men and Fatherhood in South Africa.* South Africa: HSRC Press, 13–25.

Morrell, R., Dunkle, K., Ibragimov, U. and Jewkes, R. (2016) Fathers who care and those that don't: men and childcare in South Africa, *South African Review of Sociology*, 47 (4): 80–105.

Morris, K., Featherstone, B., Hill, K. and Ward, M. (2017). *'Stepping Up, Stepping Down': How Families Make Sense of Working with Welfare Services*, Report, www.basw.co.uk/resources/stepping-stepping-down

Morris, K., Mason, W., Bywaters, P., Featherstone, B., Daniel, B., Brady, G., Bunting L., Hooper, J., Mirza, N., Scourfield, J. and Webb, C. (2018) Social work, poverty, and child welfare interventions, *Child and Family Social Work*, 23 (3): 364–372.

Murray, C. (1984) *Losing Ground: American Social Policy 1950–1980*. New York: Basic Books.

Mynarska, M., Riederer, B., Jaschinski, I., Krivanek, D., Neyer, G. and Oláh, L. (2015) *Vulnerability of Families with Children: Major Risks, Future Challenges and Policy Recommendations*, Families and Societies Working Paper No 49, www.familiesandsocieties.eu/wp-content/uploads/2015/11/WP49MynarskaEtAl2015.pdf

Naldini, M., Satta, C. and Ghigi, R. (2018) Doing family through gender, doing gender through family. Exploring social inequalities and cultural changes in everyday parenting. An introduction, *Sociologica*, 12 (3): 1–10.

Natalier, K. and Hewitt, B. (2010) 'It's not just about the money': non-resident fathers' perspectives on paying child support, *Sociology*, 44 (3): 489–505.

Natalier, K. and Hewitt, B. (2014) Separated parents reproducing and undoing gender through defining legitimate uses of child support, *Gender and Society*, 28 (6): 904–925.

Nayak, A. (2006) Displaced masculinities: chavs, youth and class in the post-industrial city, *Sociology*, 40 (5): 813–831.

Neale, B. (2000) *Theorising Family, Kinship and Social Change*, Workshop Paper No 6, Prepared for Workshop Two: Statistics and Theories for Understanding Social Change, www.leeds.ac.uk/cava/papers/wsp6.pdf

Neale, B. (2016) Introduction: young fatherhood: lived experiences and policy challenges, *Social Policy and Society*, 15 (1): 75–83.

Neale, B. (2019) *What Is Qualitative Longitudinal Research?* London: Bloomsbury.

Neale, B. (2021) *The Craft of Qualitative Longitudinal Research*. London: Sage.

Neale, B. and Davies, L. (2015a) Becoming a young breadwinner? The education, employment and training trajectories of young fathers, *Social Policy and Society*, 15 (1): 85–98.

Neale, B. and Davies, L. (2015b) *Hard to Reach? Re-thinking Support for Young Fathers*, Briefing Paper No 6, https://followingfathers.leeds.ac.uk/wp-content/uploads/sites/79/2015/10/Brieifing-Paper-6-V7.pdf

Neale, B. and Flowerdew, J. (2003) Time, texture and childhood: the contours of longitudinal qualitative research, *International Journal of Social Research Methodology*, 6 (3): 189–199.

Neale, B. and Holland, J. (2012) Researching lives through time: an introduction to the Timescapes approach, *Qualitative Research*, 12 (1): 4–15.

Neale, B. and Ladlow, L. (2015) *Finding a Place to Parent? Housing Young Fathers*, Following Young Fathers Briefing Paper No 7, https://followingfathers.leeds.ac.uk/wp-content/uploads/sites/79/2015/10/Brieifing-Paper-7-V3.pdf

Neale, B. and Patrick, R. (2016) *Engaged young fathers? Gender, parenthood and the dynamics of relationships*, Following Young Fathers Working Paper Series No 1, https://followingfathers.leeds.ac.uk/wp-content/uploads/sites/79/2015/10/FYF-Working-Paper-Engaged-young-fathers.pdf

Neale, B., Lau Clayton, C., Davies, L. and Ladlow, L. (2015) *Researching the lives of young fathers: the Following Young Fathers study and dataset*, Briefing Paper No 8, https://followingfathers.leeds.ac.uk/wp-content/uploads/sites/79/2015/10/Researching-the-Lives-of-Young-Fathers-updated-Oct-22.pdf

Neysmith, S.M., Reitsma-Street, M., Baker-Collins, S., Porter, E. and Tam, S. (2010) Provisioning responsibilities: how relationships shape the work that women do, *Canadian Review of Sociology/Revue Canadienne de Sociologie*, 47 (2): 149–170.

Nilsen, A. and Brannen, J. (2014) An intergenerational approach to transitions to adulthood: the importance of history and biography, *Sociological Research Online*, 19 (2): 1–10.

Nilsen, A. (2014) Cohort and generation: concepts in studies of social change from a life course perspective, *Families, Relationships and Societies*, 3 (3): 475–479.

Nomaguchi, K. and Johnson, W. (2014) Parenting stress among low-income and working-class fathers: the role of employment, *Journal of Family Issues*, 37 (11): 1535–1557.

Norman, H., Elliot, M. and Fagan, C. (2018) Does fathers' involvement in childcare and housework affect couples' relationship stability? *Social Science Quarterly*, 99 (5): 1599–1613.

O'Brien, M. (2011) Fathers in challenging family contexts: a need for engagement. In: United Nations (2011) *Men in Families and Family Policy in a Changing World*, www.un.org/esa/socdev/family/docs/men-in-families.pdf

O'Neill, M. and Roberts, B. (2019) *Walking Methods: Research on the Move*. Abingdon: Routledge.

Offer, S. (2012) The burden of reciprocity: processes of exclusion and withdrawal from personal networks among low-income families, *Current Sociology*, 60 (6): 788–805.

Office for National Statistics (2019) Families and Households, www.ons.gov.uk/peoplepopulationandcommunity/birthsdeathsandmarriages/families/datasets/familiesandhouseholdsfamiliesandhouseholds

Oláh, L., Richter, R. and Kotowska, I. (2018) The new roles of men and women and implications for families and societies. In: G. Doblhammer and J. Gumà (eds), *A Demographic Perspective on Gender, Family and Health in Europe*, London: Springer Link, pp 41–64.

Olchawski, J. (2016) *Parents, Work and Care: Striking the Balance*. London: Fawcett Society, www.fawcettsociety.org.uk/wp-content/uploads/2016/03/Parents-Work-andCare-2016.pdf

Parsons, T. (1954) *Essays in Sociological Theory*. New York: The Free Press.

Patrick, R. (2015) *Rhetoric and Reality: Exploring Lived Experiences of Welfare Reform under the Coalition*. Social Policy Association: What's the point of welfare? Series, www.social-policy.org.uk/wordpress/wp-content/uploads/2015/04/06_patrick.pdf

Patrick, R., Garthwaite, K. and Power, M. (2020) Researching COVID-19 and its impact on families: some ethical challenges, *Discover Society*, https://discoversociety.org/2020/04/23/researching-covid-19-and-its-impact-on-families-some-ethical-challenges/

Philip, G., Clifton, J. and Brandon, M. (2018) The trouble with fathers: the impact of time and gendered-thinking on working relationships between fathers and social workers in child protection practice in England, *Journal of Family Issues*, 40 (6): 2288–2309.

Philip, G., Youansamouth, L., Bedston, S., Broadhurst, K., Hu, Y., Clifton, J. and Brandon, M. (2020) 'I had no hope, I had no help at all': insights from a first study of fathers and recurrent care proceedings, *Societies*, 10 (4): 89–105.

Pilcher, J., Williams, J. and Pole, C. (2003) Rethinking adulthood: families, transitions, and social change, *Sociological Research Online*, 8 (4): 181–185.

Plantin, L., Mansson, S. and Kearney, J. (2003) Talking and doing fatherhood: on fatherhood and masculinity in Sweden and England, *Fathering*, 1 (1): 3–26.

Poole, E., Speight, S., O'Brien, M., Connolly, S. and Aldrich, M. (2016) Who are non-resident fathers? A British socio-demographic profile, *Journal of Social Policy*, 45 (2): 223–250.

Power, A. and Hall, E. (2017) Placing care in times of austerity, *Social and Cultural Geography*, 19 (3): 303–313.

Power, M., Patrick, R., Garthwaite, K. and Page, G. (2020) COVID realities: everyday life for families on a low income during the pandemic, Briefing Paper, https://mk0nuffieldfounpg9ee.kinstacdn.com/wp-content/uploads/2020/04/Exploratory-Study-Briefing-Note.pdf

Prison Reform Trust (2013) Prison: the facts, Bromley Briefings summer report, www.prisonreformtrust.org.uk/Portals/0/Documents/Prisonthefacts.pdf

Quaid, S. (2018) Mothering in an age of austerity. In: P. Rushton and C. Donovan (eds), *Austerity Policies: Bad Ideas in Practice*. London: Springer, 67–88.

Randles, J. (2018) 'Manning up' to be a good father: hybrid fatherhood, masculinity, and US responsible fatherhood policy, *Gender and Society*, 32 (4): 516–539.

Randles, J. (2020) Role modelling responsibility: the essential father discourse, I: responsible fatherhood programming and policy, *Social Problems*, 67: 96–112.

Rao, A.H. (2020) *Crunch Time: How Married Couples Confront Unemployment*. Berkeley: University of California Press.

Reeves, J., Gale, L., Webb, J., Delaney, R. and Cocklin, N. (2009) Focusing on young men: developing integrated services for young fathers, *Community Practitioner: The Journal of the Community Practitioners' and Health Visitors' Association*, 82 (9):18.

Reynolds, T. (2009) Exploring the absent/present dilemma: Black fathers, family relationships, and social capital in Britain, *The Annals of the American Academy of Political and Social Science*, 624 (1): 12–28.

Reynolds, T. (2010) The vast majority of black children are raised in stable, loving homes, *The Guardian*, www.theguardian.com/commentisfree/2010/mar/24/vast-majority-black-boys-loving-homes

Reynolds, T. (2020) Studies of the maternal: Black mothering 10 years on, *Studies of the Maternal*, http://doi.org/10.16995/sim.290

Ribbens McCarthy, J., Edwards, R. and Gillies, V. (2003) *Making Families: Moral Tales of Parenting and Step-parenting*. Durham, NC: Sociology Press.

Richards Solomon, C. (2017) *The Lives of Stay-at-Home Fathers: Masculinity, Carework and Fatherhood in the United States.* Bingley: Emerald Publishing.

Richter, L. and Morrell, R. (2006) *BABA: Men and Fatherhood in South Africa.* South Africa: HSRC Press. 13–25.

Ridge, T. (2009) *Living with Poverty: A Review of the Literature on Children's and Families' Experiences of Poverty.* London: Department for Work and Pensions.

Ridge, T. (2013) 'We are all in this together'? The hidden costs of poverty, recession and austerity policies on Britain's poorest children, *Children and Society*, 27 (5): 406–417.

Ridge, T. and Millar, J. (2008) *Work and Wellbeing over Time: Lone Mothers and their Children.* London: Department for Work and Pensions Research Report No 536.

Robb, M. (2019) *Men, Masculinities, and the Care of Children: Images, Ideas and Identities.* Abingdon: Routledge.

Robb, M., Featherstone, B., Ruxton, S. and Ward, M.R.M. (2015) *Beyond Male Role Models, Gender Identity and Work with Young Men*, Project report, www.open.ac.uk/health-and-social-care/research/beyond-male-role-models/report

Robb, M., Featherstone, B., Ruxton, S. and Ward, M.R.M. (2018) Family relationships and troubled masculinities: the experience of young men in contact with care and welfare services. In: L. O'Dell, C. Brownlow and H. Bertilsdotter-Rosqvist (eds), *Different Childhoods: Non/Normative Development and Transgressive Trajectories.* Abingdon: Routledge: 72–84.

Roberts, S. (2013) Boys will be boys ... won't they? Change and continuities in contemporary young working-class masculinities, *Sociology*, 47: 671–686.

Roberts, S. (2014) *Debating Modern Masculinities: Change, Continuity, Crisis?* Basingstoke: Palgrave MacMillan.

Roberts, S. (2018) *Young Working-Class Men in Transition.* Abingdon: Routledge.

Roberts, S. and Elliott, K. (2020) Challenging dominant representations of marginalised boys and men in critical studies on men and masculinities, *Boyhood Studies*, 13 (2): 87–104.

Robertson, S., Woodall, J., Henry, H., Hanna, E., Rowlands, S., Horrocks, S., Livesley, J. and Long, T. (2016) Evaluating a community-led project for improving fathers' and children's wellbeing in England, *Health Promotion International*, 33 (3): 410–421.

Robinson, V. and Hockey, J. (2011) *Masculinities in Transition.* Basingstoke: Palgrave Macmillan.

Robinson, C.A., Bottorff, J.L., Pesut, B., Oliffe, J.L. and Tomlinson, J. (2014) The male face of caregiving: a scoping review of men caring for a person with dementia, *American Journal of Men's Health*, 8 (5): 409–426.

Rosenberg, J. and Wilcox, W.B. (2006) *The Importance of Fathers in the Healthy Development of Children: Fathers and Their Impact on Children's Well-Being*. U.S. Children's Bureau, Office on Child Abuse and Neglect.

Roy, K. (1999) Low-income single fathers in an African American community and the requirements of welfare reform, *Journal of Family Issues*, 20 (4): 432–457.

Roy, K. (2004) Three-Block fathers: spatial perceptions and kin-work in low-income African American neighbourhoods, *Social Problems*, 51 (4): 528–548.

Roy, K. (2006) Father stories: a life course examination of paternal identity among low-income African American men, *Journal of Family Issues*, 27 (1): 31–54.

Roy, K., Palkovitz, R. and Waters, D. (2015) Low-income fathers as resilient care-givers. In: J.A. Arditti (ed), *Family Problems: Stress, Risk, and Resilience*. Oxford: Wiley Blackwell, 83–98.

Ruxton, S. (2002) *Men, Masculinities and Poverty in the UK*. London: Oxfam.

Ruxton, S. and Burrell, S. (2020) *Masculinities and COVID-19: Making the Connections*, London: Promundo.

Scourfield, J., Yi Cheung, S. and MacDonald, G. (2014) Working with fathers to improve children's well-being: results of a survey exploring service provision and intervention approach in the UK, *Children and Youth Services Review*, 43: 40–50.

Segal, L. (1990) *Slow Motion: Changing Masculinities, Changing Men*. Basingstoke: Palgrave Macmillan.

Segal, L. (2006) *Slow Motion: Changing Masculinities, Changing Men* (3rd edn). Basingstoke: Palgrave Macmillan.

Setftersten, R.A. and Lovegreen, L.D. (1998) Educational experiences throughout adult life: new hopes or no hope for life-course flexibility? *Research on Aging*, 20 (4): 506–538.

Sewell, T. (2019) Rod Liddle is right about black boys and absent dads, *The Spectator*, www.spectator.co.uk/article/rod-liddle-is-right-about-black-boys-and-absent-dads

Shildrick, T. (2018) *Poverty Propaganda: Exploring the Myths*. Bristol: Policy Press.

Shildrick, T., MacDonald, R., Webster, C. and Garthwaite, K. (2012) *Poverty and Insecurity: Life in Low-Pay, No-Pay Britain.* Bristol: Policy Press.

Shirani, F., Henwood, K. and Coltart, C. (2012) 'Why aren't you in work?' Negotiating economic models of fathering identity, *Fathering*, 10 (3): 274–290.

Shows, C. and Gerstel, N. (2009) Fathering, class, and gender: a comparison of physicians and emergency medical technicians, *Gender and Society*, 23 (2): 161–187.

Silva, E. and Smart, C. (1997) *The New Family?* London: Sage.

Simpson, P. and Richards, M. (2019) Reflexivity denied? The emotional and health-seeking resources of men facing disadvantage, *Sociology of Health and Illness*, 41 (5): 900–916.

Skevik, A. (2006) 'Absent fathers' or 'reorganized families'? Variations in father–child contact after parental break-up in Norway, *The Sociological Review*, 54 (1): 114–132.

Slutskaya, N., Simson, R., Hughes, J., Simpson, A. and Uygur, S. (2016) Masculinity and class in the context of dirty work, *Gender, Work and Organisation*, 23 (2): 165–182.

Smart, C. (2007) *Personal Life.* Cambridge: Polity Press.

Smart, C. and Neale, B. (1999) 'I hadn't really thought about it': new identities/new fatherhoods. In: J. Seymour and P. Bagguley (eds), *Relating Intimacies: Power and Resistance.* London: Springer: 118–141.

Smith, J.A. (2009) *The Daddy Shift: How Stay-at-Home Dads, Breadwinning Moms, and Shared Parenting are Transforming the American Family.* Boston, MA: Beacon Press.

Smith, N.D. and Middleton, S. (2009) *A Review of Poverty Dynamics Research in the UK.* York: Joseph Rowntree Foundation.

Smooth, W.G. (2013) Intersectionality from theoretical framework to policy intervention. In: A.R. Wilson (ed), *Situating Intersectionality.* London: Springer.

Stacey, J. (1998) Dads-ism in the 1990s: getting past baby talk about fatherlessness. In: C.R. Daniels (ed), *Lost Fathers: The Politics of Fatherlessness in America.* New York: St Martin's Griffin.

Stack, C. (1974) *All Our Kin: Strategies for Survival in a Black Community.* New York: Basic Books.

Strange, J.M. (2012) Fatherhood, providing, and attachment in late Victorian and Edwardian working-class families, *The Historical Journal*, 55 (4): 1007–1027.

Strange, J.M. (2015) *Fatherhood and the British Working Class, 1865–1914.* Cambridge: Cambridge University Press.

Strier, R. (2014) Unemployment and fatherhood: gender, culture and national context, *Gender, Work and Organisation*, 21 (5): 395–410.

Strier, R., Eiskovits, Z., Sigad, L. and Buchbinder, E. (2014) Masculinity, poverty and work: the multiple construction of work among working poor men, *Journal of Social Policy*, 43: 331–349.

Summers, J.A., Boller, K., Schiffman, R.F. and Raikes, H.H. (2006) The Meaning of "Good Fatherhood:" Low-Income Fathers' Social Constructions of Their Roles, *Parenting*, 6 (2-3): 145-165.

Tarrant, A. (2013) Grandfathering as spatio-temporal practice: conceptualizing performances of ageing masculinities in contemporary familial carescapes, *Social and Cultural Geography*, 14 (2): 192–210.

Tarrant, A. (2015) *Stakeholder Meeting: Men, Poverty and Lifetimes of Care Research Project*, Report, https://cpb-eu-w2.wpmucdn.com/blogs. lincoln.ac.uk/dist/e/6201/files/2016/11/Stakeholder-Meeting-Report-for-stakeholders.pdf

Tarrant, A. (2017) Getting out of the swamp? Methodological reflections on using qualitative secondary analysis to develop research design, *International Journal of Social Research Methodology*, 20 (6): 599–611.

Tarrant, A. (2018) Care in an age of austerity: men's care responsibilities in low-income families, *Ethics and Social Welfare*, 12 (1): 34–48.

Tarrant, A. (2021) Austerity and men's hidden family participation in low-income families in the UK. In: S.-M. Hall, H. Pimlott-Wilson and J. Horton (eds), *Austerity across Europe: Lived Experiences of Economic Crises*. Abingdon: Routledge.

Tarrant, A. and Hughes, K. (2019) Qualitative secondary analysis: building longitudinal samples to understand men's generational identities in low income contexts, *Sociology*, 53 (3) 538–553.

Tarrant, A. and Hughes, K. (2020) The ethics of technology choice: photovoice methodology with men living in low-income contexts, *Sociological Research Online*, 25 (2): 289–306.

Tarrant, A. and Neale, B. (2017a) *Learning to Support Young Dads*, Responding to Young Fathers in a Different Way: Project Report, https://followingfathers.leeds.ac.uk/wp-content/uploads/sites/79/ 2017/04/SYD-final-report.pdf

Tarrant, A. and Neale, B. (2017b) *Supporting Young Fathers in Welfare Settings: An Evidence Review of What Matters and What Helps*, Responding to Young Fathers in a Different Way: Evidence Review, https://followingfathers.leeds.ac.uk/wp-content/uploads/sites/79/ 2016/06/Evidence-Report.pdf

Tarrant, A. and Ward, M. (2017) The myth of the fatherless society, *The Conversation*, https://theconversation.com/the-myth-of-the-fatherless-society-73166

Tarrant, A., Way, L. and Ladlow, L. (2020a) *Negotiating 'Earning' and 'Caring' through the COVID-19 Crisis: Change and Continuities in the Parenting and Employment Trajectories of Young Fathers*, https://docs.google.com/viewerng/viewer?url=https://fyff.blogs.lincoln.ac.uk/files/2020/12/COVID-19-FYFF-Briefing-Paper-One-FINAL.pdf&hl=en

Tarrant, A., Ladlow, L. and Way, L. (2020b) *From Social Isolation to Local Support: Relational Change and Continuities for Young Fathers in the Context of the COVID 19 Crisis*, https://docs.google.com/viewerng/viewer?url=https://fyff.blogs.lincoln.ac.uk/files/2020/12/COVID-19-FYFF-Briefing-Paper-One-FINAL.pdf&hl=en

Tarrant, A., Terry, G., Ward, M.R., Ruxton, S., Robb, M. and Featherstone, B. (2015) Are male role models really the solution? Interrogating the 'war on boys' through the lens of the 'male role model' discourse, *Boyhood Studies*, 8 (1): 60–83.

Tarrant, A., Featherstone, B., O'Dell, L. and Fraser, C. (2017) 'You try to keep a brave face on but inside you are in bits': grandparent experiences of engaging with professionals in children's services, *Qualitative Social Work*, 16 (3): 351–366.

Timonen, V. (2020) *Grandparenting Practices around the World: Reshaping Family*. Bristol: Policy Press.

Tosh, J. (1996) Authority and nurture in middle-class fatherhood: the case of early and mid-Victorian England, *Gender and History*, 8 (1) 48–64.

Tosh, J. (1999) *A Man's Place: Masculinity and the Middle-Class Home in Victorian England*. New Haven: Yale University Press.

Townsend, N. (2002) *Package Deal: Marriage, Work and Fatherhood in Men's Lives*. Philadelphia: Temple University Press.

Tronto, J.C. (1993) *Moral Boundaries: A Political Argument for an Ethic of Care*. Abingdon: Routledge.

Tyler, I. (2008) "Chav mum chav scum": class disgust in contemporary Britain, *Feminist Media Studies*, 8 (1): 17–34.

Tyler, I. (2013) The riots of the underclass? Stigmatisation, mediation and the government of poverty and disadvantage in neoliberal Britain, *Sociological Research Online*, 18 (4): 6.

United Nations (2011) *Men in Families and Family Policy in a Changing World*, www.un.org/esa/socdev/family/docs/men-in-families.pdf

van der Gaag, N., Heilman, B., Gupta, T., Nembhard, C. and Barker, G. (2019) *State of the World's Fathers: Unlocking the Power of Men's Care: Executive Summary*. Washington, DC: Promundo-US.

van der Heijden, K., Visse, M., Lensvelt-Mulders, G. and Widdershoven, G. (2016) To care or not to care? A narrative on experiencing caring responsibilities, *Ethics and Social Welfare*, 10 (1): 53–68.

Wacquant, L. (2008a) Territorial stigmatization in the age of advanced marginality. In: J. Houtsonen and A. Antikainen (eds), *Symbolic Power in Cultural Contexts*. Leiden: Brill Sense, 43–52.

Wacquant, L. (2008b) *Urban Outcasts: A Comparative Sociology of Advanced Marginality*. Cambridge: Polity Press.

Wacquant, L. (2010) Crafting the neoliberal state: workfare, prisonfare, and social insecurity, *Sociological Forum*, 25 (2): 197–220.

Wacquant, L., Slater, T. and Pereira, V. (2014) Territorial stigmatization in action, *Environment and Planning A*, 46 (6): 1270–1280.

Walker, C. and Roberts, S. (2018) *Masculinity, Labour, and Neoliberalism: Working-class Men in International Perspective*. Basingstoke: Palgrave Macmillan.

Walker, G.W. (2006) Disciplining protest masculinity, *Men and Masculinities*, 9 (1): 5–22.

Walklate, S. (2007) *Imagining the Victim of Crime*. Buckingham: Open University Press.

Waller, M.R. (2002) *My Baby's Father: Unmarried Parents and Paternal Responsibility*. Ithaca, NY: Cornell University Press.

Ward, M.R.M. (2015a) *From Labouring to Learning: Working-Class Masculinities, Education and De-Industrialization*. Basingstoke: Palgrave Macmillan.

Ward, M.R.M. (2015b) The chameleonisation of masculinity: Jimmy's multiple performances of a working-class self. *Masculinities and Social Change*, 4 (3): 215–240.

Ward, M.R.M. (2020) Men, masculinities and social class. In: L. Gottsen, U. Mellstrom and T. Shefer (eds), *International Handbook of Masculinity Studies*. London: Routledge.

Ward, M.R.M., Tarrant, A., Terry, G., Featherstone, B., Robb, M. and Ruxton, S. (2017) Doing gender locally: the importance of 'place' in understanding marginalised masculinities and young men's transitions to 'safe' and successful futures, *The Sociological Review*, 65 (4): 797–815.

Warren, J. (2017) *Industrial Teesside, Lives and Legacies: A Post-industrial Geography*. Basingstoke: Palgrave Macmillan.

Washbrook, E. (2007) *Fathers, Childcare and Children's Readiness to Learn*, The Centre for Market and Public Organisation, Working Paper No. 07/175, University of Bristol.

Watt, P. (2020) Territorial stigmatisation and poor housing at a London 'sink estate', *Social Inclusion*, 8 (1): 20–33.

Webster, C., Simpson, D. and MacDonald, R. (2004) *Poor Transitions: Social Exclusion and Young Adults*. Bristol: Policy Press.

Welfare Conditionality Project (2018) *Welfare Conditionality Report 2013–2018: Final Findings*, www.welfareconditionality.ac.uk/publications/final-findings-welcond-project/

Wellard, S. (2012) Older people as grandparents: how public policy needs to broaden its view of older people and the role they play within families, *Quality in Ageing and Older Adults*, 13 (4): 257–263.

Welshman, J. (2012) *From Transmitted Deprivation to Social Exclusion: Policy, Poverty and Parenting*. Bristol: Policy Press.

Welshman, J. (2013) Troubles and the family: changes and continuities since 1943, *Social Policy and Society*, 16 (1): 109–117.

West, C. and Zimmerman (1987) Doing gender, *Gender and Society*, 1 (2): 125–151.

Whitehead, S.M. (2002) *Men and Masculinities: Key Themes and New Directions*. Cambridge: Polity Press.

Williams, F. (1998) Troubled masculinities in social policy discourses: fatherhood. In: J. Popay, J. Hearn and J. Edwards (eds), *Men, Gender Divisions and Welfare*. Abingdon: Routledge, 63–100.

Williams, F. (2004) *Rethinking Families*. Lisbon: Calouste Gulbenkian Foundation.

Williams, J. (2010) *Reshaping the Work–Family Debate: Why Men and Class Matter*. Cambridge, MA: Harvard University Press.

Williams, R.A. (2009) Masculinities and fathering, *Community, Work and Family*, 12 (1): 57–73.

Willott, S. and Griffin, C. (1997) 'Wham bam, am I a man?' Unemployed men talk about masculinities, *Feminism and Psychology*, 7 (1) 107–128.

Wissö, T. (2018) Researching fatherhood and place: adopting an ethnographic approach. In: E. Dermott and C. Gatrell (eds), *Fathers, Families and Relationships: Researching Everyday Lives*. Bristol: Policy Press. 89–108.

Women's Budget Group (2018) *The Impact of Austerity on Women in the UK*, www.ohchr.org/Documents/Issues/Development/IEDebt/WomenAusterity/WBG.pdf

Working Families (2017) *Working Families Index 2017*, www.workingfamilies.org.uk/wp-content/uploads/2017/01/Modern-Families-Index_Full-Report-1.pdfModern

Yarwood, G.A. (2011) The pick and mix of fathering identities, *Fathering*, 9: 150–168.

Yeandle, S., Escott, K., Grant, L. and Batty, E. (2003) *Women and Men Talking about Poverty*, Working Paper series No 7. Manchester: Equal Opportunities Commission.

Young, M. and Willmott, P. (1978) *Family and Kinship in East London* (rev. edn). London: Penguin Books.

Zanoni, L., Warburton, W., Bussey, K and McMaugh, A. (2013) Fathers as 'core business' in child welfare practice and research, *Children and Youth Services*, 35: 1055–1070.

Index